I0134954

30/30 Fitness

Thirty, thirty-minute easy home workouts for improving your health and wellbeing

MARIANNE GATES

Illustrated by Pauline Mumford

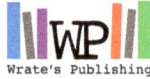

![Wrate's Publishing logo] WP Wrate's Publishing

First published 2020 by Wrate's Publishing

ISBN 978-1-8380128-9-2

Copyright © Marianne Gates

Edited and typeset by Wrate's Editing Services
www.wrateseditingservices.co.uk

To my father, Brian Colin Gates (5th March 1950 – 23rd April 2020)

The right of Marianne Gates to be identified as the author of this work has been asserted in accordance with the Copyright, Designs and Patents Act, 1988.

All rights reserved. No part of this publication may be reproduced, stored in a retrieval system, or transmitted, in any form or by any means (electronic, mechanical, photocopying, recording or otherwise), without the prior written permission of the publisher.

A CIP catalogue record for this book is available from the British Library.

Contents

Introduction

As a competitive athlete and qualified personal trainer, it's no great coincidence that most of my friends, colleagues and social media acquaintances are involved in the fitness industry. This isn't a bad thing, as we learn from, motivate and push each other to work harder to achieve our goals. Many of my exercise enthusiastic friends are also social media influencers and post and share their workouts on a daily basis. And here's where I have noticed a trend. Many of these programmes are designed for people with advanced fitness levels and involve complex movements, weighted exercises and sessions that are time consuming as well as being complicated to follow and perform. It became apparent to me that the majority of us fitness instructors, especially the ones hoping to attract a large social media following, have forgotten about the 'normal people', who may just want to become more active and improve their health without necessarily being able to do a thousand burpees or run a marathon. Their goal might be simply to reserve thirty minutes or so from their day to move their bodies. And I would encourage everyone to do this. Being active for just half an hour a day has a positive impact on the mind, body and soul. It will also help to reduce your chances of succumbing to illness and injury.

With this in mind, I decided to compile a series of routines that you can do over 30 minutes in your day, for 30 days (these don't have to be consecutive). They can be done any time, any place, anywhere, and they are easy to understand and follow. Moreover, you don't need to be a fitness buff to join in and can be any age, shape or size!

Who is this book aimed at?

These exercises would work for you if you fall into one or more of these categories. You typically:

- Feel nervous at the thought of starting a new exercise regimen.

- Have looked on the internet but are daunted or confused by what you've found. You don't know where to start or which programme to choose.

- Find going to the gym or joining in exercise classes scary and intimidating.

- Can't afford gym membership or have no access to a gym or fitness studio.

- Don't have a lot of free time in which to exercise.

My story

My name is Marianne Gates, I am 43 years old and I currently reside in China with my husband. I haven't always worked in the fitness industry. Originally from South Africa, I studied Nuclear Medicine and had a career within this field for the best part of a decade. My job took me all over the world, and I have also lived in Saudi Arabia, Dubai and the UK.

Back when I was a student, my life now would have been unimaginable to me. At both school and college, I was more academically orientated, and sport simply wasn't on my radar. I was overweight by 22 to 33lbs (10-15kg) and was not given the opportunity to develop at a sporting level. At school, the teachers only really focused on the students who were gifted athletes. Although I wasn't bad at swimming, I wasn't at a level to be noticed and my weight issues meant I was self-conscious about wearing my swimsuit in public. My early experiences gave me an insight into what it's like not to feel natural or confident when it comes to sport, which helps me to help clients who may also have formed the impression that for whatever reason, exercise just isn't for them.

My passion for sport and exercise only came to the fore when I was in my mid-twenties. My father suffered a severe angina attack (resulting from blocked coronary arteries) and he was diagnosed with high cholesterol. As this can be hereditary, and as I was also still carrying excess weight, I decided to have my own cholesterol tested. The results came back revealing a high level for my age group. This is when I made the conscious decision to eat more healthily and take daily exercise. I started by going for walks and then, with the encouragement of my friends, I joined a gym and started weight training. As my confidence grew, I signed up for circuit and spinning classes and the rest, as they say, is history.

Fast forward to 2014, and I was given the opportunity to focus on my training and sport. With this extra time, I decided to retrain as a Personal Trainer and Hatha Yoga Instructor. I have mainly worked with clients in boutique gyms. I am always reading and aspiring to gain more knowledge about different training methods, and my next goal is to focus on sports therapy and study traditional Chinese medicine as an alternative method to help athletes recover from injury.

My journey to competitive fitness

In 2010, my husband and I relocated to Dubai. In the hope of making some new friends, I joined a local gym (exercising indoors is also essential during the summer in Dubai, where temperatures can reach 50 Celsius plus). It was one of my new gym friends who invited me to run the Dubai Marathon with her. I was truly shocked that she thought I'd be up to such a long-distance run, but with the encouragement of my husband, I decided to sign up. This proved a catalyst, and several marathons and half-marathons followed. Around the same time, I also developed an interest (some might say obsession, oops) in CrossFit, a strength, conditioning and overall fitness programme that is also a competitive sport and incorporates elements from practices including high-intensity interval training, Olympic weightlifting and gymnastics. This led me to competing in the Dubai Fitness Championship in 2014, 2015 and 2016. In 2014, I also qualified as an individual competitor from the Middle East region to take part in the CrossFit Asia Regionals, held in South Korea. As this is an extremely challenging competition, I decided to get involved as part of a team, as this way I could share the workload and my teammates and I could support each other. It was a truly life-changing experience. Little old me, who never got to join in with sports at school, was suddenly competing against some of the top teams in the CrossFit field. This was a major boost to my confidence and self-esteem.

Soon after this, another group of friends, who were training for the Dubai International Triathlon, invited me to join them. Doubting my ability once again, I mentioned it to my husband, whose response was, 'You can do it, go for it!' This led me to compete in several Half Iron Man Races, where you cover a distance of 70.3 miles in total, comprising a 1.2-mile (1.9 km) swim, a 56-mile (90 km) bike ride and a 13.1-mile (21.1 km) run. So far, I have participated in three 70.3-mile world championships, in Australia, America and South Africa.

As well as taking part in triathlons, I have also started running ultramarathons (any race that is longer than a traditional marathon length of 26.2 miles or 42.195 km) and love the mental challenge of completing these really long runs. My longest run so far has been 44.74 miles (72 km), which I completed in the Sultanate of Oman.

Training for triathlons and ultramarathons is really hard and time consuming, but crossing the finishing line is an amazing feeling that I find hard to put into words. I truly feel blessed to have the opportunity to compete in these events, as well as for having an amazing husband who champions my crazy adventures.

On a personal note

I wish to stress again that I don't come from an athletic background, I have simply learned and practised different exercise methods over the years and found what works for me through trial and error. I love helping people realise they can get fitter regardless of their current size, age, weight or any mental blocks they may carry. I used to have a deeply embedded 'I can't' mindset, which I gradually managed to change to an 'I can' one. Whatever your goal, my aim is to help you change your mindset, too. You can do it!

Disclaimer

Before we go further, I need to add that I am not your doctor, nor do I have the opportunity to see you personally. If at any time you feel a high degree of discomfort during an exercise, then stop and consult a medical practitioner. Depending on your level of activity before starting an exercise programme, it's often a good idea to have a physical examination in order to set a baseline for a review in the future.

How to use this book

I have put together 30, 30-minute workouts, running from Day 1 to Day 30. You'll find these listed in the table (starting on page 14), along with the page number for each exercise, which is illustrated as well as described, making it simple for you to follow.

The exercises are separated into four different groups, depending on which area of the body they target: Upper Body, Lower Body, Core (abdominals and back) and overall Metabolic Conditioning. (Metabolic Conditioning exercises vary from moderate to high intensity. Their purpose is to improve both your aerobic – with oxygen – and anaerobic – without – cardiovascular systems.)

In addition, the exercises are colour-coded (see the key) to help you easily find ones from a particular group. The group each exercise falls into is also listed in the table in brackets.

Keep in mind that each routine is only a guide and the exercises can be mixed and matched. Nor do the routines have to be performed consecutively. A good practice would be to complete a different routine for two or three days in a row before taking a day off.

I have designed the workouts so they can be performed in limited space with little or no equipment, which means they will be easy to fit around your current lifestyle. They will also benefit your entire body. I advise keeping a diary as you follow the programme, so you can note down the improvements to your fitness and wellbeing and tweak the routines (if necessary) to suit your own preferences (this is when the colour-coding will really help) when you begin the cycle again. Please have fun and enjoy your journey to a fitter you.

KEY TO COLOURS AND TABS	
UPPER BODY	Upper Body (UB)
LOWER BODY	Lower Body (LB)
METABOLIC CONDITIONING	Metabolic Conditioning (MC)
CORE/ABS/ BACK	Core/Abs/Back (CAB)

The Routines
(by day)

Aim for 3-6 rounds and 8-20 repetitions per movement. A short warm-up can be done by performing 3-5 repetitions of each movement in the routine. This will get your body prepped for the movements to follow and you will also become familiar with the exercises.

DAY 1	DAY 2	DAY 3
Lunges (LB) Page 36	Sumo squats (LB) Page 39	Glute bridges (LB) Page 40
Squats (LB) Page 35	Inch worms (UB) Page 25	Plank shoulder taps (UB, CAB) Page 28, 72
Push-ups (UB) Page 22-24	Crunches straight into leg raises (CAB) Page 62, 63	Lunges (LB) Page 6
Plank on forearms (UB, CAB) Page 27, 71	Plank toe taps (UB, CAB) Page 29, 73	Bird dog (LB) Page 43
Burpees (MC) Page 47-48	Mountain climbers (UB, MC) (Aim for a fast pace in order to maximise the cardiovascular benefit.) Page 32, 54	In-and-out running on the spot (MC) (Simulating sprinting on the spot.) Page 53

Day 4	Day 5	Day 6
Frog hops (MC) Page 60	Side lunges (LB) Page 37	Squats (LB) Page 35
Bicycles (CAB) Page 65	Bird dog (LB) Page 43	Fire hydrants (LB) Page 42
Plank walkouts (CAB) Page 74	Curtsy lunges (LB) Page 45	Crunches straight into Russian twists (CAB) Page 62, 77-78
Crab walks (or glute bridges on page 40, if space is limited) (UB, MC) Page 34, 57	Sit-ups (CAB) Page 61	Dips (UB) Page 30-31
Heel flicks (MC) Page 52	Side hops (MC) Page 59	In-and-out running on the spot (MC) Page 53
Day 7	**Day 8**	**Day 9**
High plank (UB, CAB) Page 26, 70	Curtsy lunges (LB) Page 45	Squat hops (MC) Page 55
Side plank (CAB) Page 75-76	Crunches (CAB) Page 62	Crab walks (or glute bridges on page 40, if space is limited) (UB, MC) Page 34, 57
Squats (LB) Page 35	Reverse lunge high knee (LB) Page 46	Bear crawls (or burpees if space is limited, page 47) (UB, LB, MC) Page 33, 44, 56
Side lunges (LB) Page 37	Sit-ups (CAB) Page 61	Side plank (CAB) Page 75-76
Jumping jacks (MC) Page 49-50	Mountain climbers (Aim for a fast pace to get a cardiovascular stimulus.) (UB, MC) Page 32, 54	V-ups (Remember that quality movements are more valuable than complex movements when your body is not ready.) (CAB) Page 68

Day 10	Day 11	Day 12
Inch worms (UB) Page 25	Superman (CAB) Page 79	Bulgarian split squats (LB) Page 41
Reverse lunge high knee (LB) Page 46	Plank shoulder taps (UB, CAB) Page 28, 72	Leg raises (Double or single leg.) (CAB) Page 63-64
Push-ups (UB) Page 22-24	Dips (UB) Page 30-31	Lunges (LB) Page 36
Sumo squats (LB) Page 39	Squats (LB) Page 35	Inch worms (UB) Page 25
Heel flicks (MC) Page 52	High knees (Aim for fast action knees.) (MC) Page 51	In-and-out running on the spot (MC) Page 53

Day 13	Day 14	Day 15
Push-ups (UB) Page 22-24	Curtsy lunges (LB) Page 45	Lunges (LB) Page 36
Side lunges (LB) Page 37	Russian twists (CAB) Page 77-78	Leg raises straight into scissors (CAB) Page 63, 67
High plank (UB, CAB) Page 26, 70	Plank walks (CAB) Page 74	Frog hops (MC) Page 60
Sumo squats (LB) Page 39	Crunches (CAB) Page 62	Push-ups (UB) Page 22-24
Skaters (MC) Page 58	Burpees (MC) Page 47-48	Jumping jacks (MC) Page 49-50

Day 16	Day 17	Day 18
Fire hydrants (LB) Page 42	Dips (UB) Page 30-31	Squats (LB) Page 35
Sit-ups (CAB) Page 61	Plank shoulder taps (UB, CAB) Page 28, 72	Inch worms (UB) Page 25
Mountain climbers (These are performed in a slow and controlled manner, focusing on your abdominals.) (UB, MC) Page 32, 54	Bird dog (LB) Page 43	Push-ups (UB) Page 22-24
Russian twists (CAB) Page 77-78	Superman (CAB) Page 79	Reverse lunge high knee (LB) Page 46
Side hops (MC) Page 59	Skaters (MC) Page 58	Bear crawls (or burpees if space is limited, page 47-48) (UB, LB, MC) Page 33, 44, 56
Day 19	**Day 20**	**Day 21**
Leg raises (Double or single leg.) (CAB) Page 63-64	Sumo squats (LB) Page 39	Bulgarian split squats (LB) Page 41
Curtsy lunges (LB) Page 45	Inch worms (UB) Page 25	Lunges (LB) Page 36
Sit-ups straight into crunches (CAB) Page 61-62	Good mornings (LB) Page 38	V-ups or single leg V-ups (CAB) Page 68, 69
Glute bridges (LB) Page 40	Dips (UB) Page 30-31	Squats (LB) Page 35
Burpees (MC) Page 47-48	High knees (if space is limited, in-and-out running on the spot) (MC) Page 51, 53	Burpees (MC) Page 47-48

Day 22	Day 23	Day 24
Plank shoulder taps (UB, CAB) Page 28, 72	Squats (LB) Page 35	Plank toe taps (UB, CAB) Page 29, 73
Burpees (MC) Page 47-48	Glute bridges (LB) Page 40	Bird dogs straight into fire hydrants (LB) Page 43, 42
Plank toe taps (UB, CAB) Page 29, 73	Side lunges (LB) Page 37	V-ups or single leg V-ups (CAB) Page 68, 69
Reverse lunge high knee (LB) Page 46	Crunches straight into leg raises (CAB) Page 62, 63	Sit-ups (CAB) Page 61
Jumping jacks (MC) Page 49-50	Mountain climbers (fast pace) (UB, MC) Page 32, 54	In-and-out running on the spot (MC) Page 53
Day 25	Day 26	Day 27
Side lunges (LB) Page 37	Inch worms (UB) Page 25	Burpees (MC) Page 47-48
Seated knee tucks (CAB) Page 66	Reverse lunge high knee (LB) Page 46	Lunges (LB) Page 36
Bulgarian split squats (LB) Page 41	Plank toe taps (UB, CAB) Page 29, 73	In-and-out running on the spot (MC) Page 53
Scissor kicks (CAB) Page 67	Superman (CAB) Page 79	Squats (LB) Page 35
Burpees (MC) Page 47-48	Heel flicks (MC) Page 52	High knees (MC) Page 51

Day 28	Day 29	Day 30
Sit-ups (CAB) Page 61	Curtsy lunges (LB) Page 45	Push-ups (UB) Page 22-24
Bulgarian split squats (LB) Page 41	Plank walks (CAB) Page 74	Lunges (LB) Page 36
Crunches straight into leg raises (CAB) Page 62, 63	Frog hops (MC) Page 60	Dips (UB) Page 30-31
Glute bridges (LB) Page 40	Crunches (CAB) Page 62	Squats (LB) Page 35
Skaters (MC) Page 58	High knees (if space is limited, in-and-out running on the spot) (MC) Page 51, 53	Burpees (MC) Page 47-48

Movement Glossary

Upper Body

Push-Up

Push-ups exercise the chest, shoulders, arms and core muscles (abdominals, back and glutes).

Begin at the top of the movement, keeping your body rigid and straight. With your hands slightly wider apart than your shoulders, keep your core activated (squeeze your glutes/buttocks, ensure your abs are tight and your naval is drawn in towards the spine) and lower your body until your chest touches the floor (bottom of the movement). Now forcefully press up through your hands, keeping your body in a straight line and returning to the start position (top of the movement). This is one repetition and should be a fluid motion, with your shoulder, core and leg muscles activated throughout.

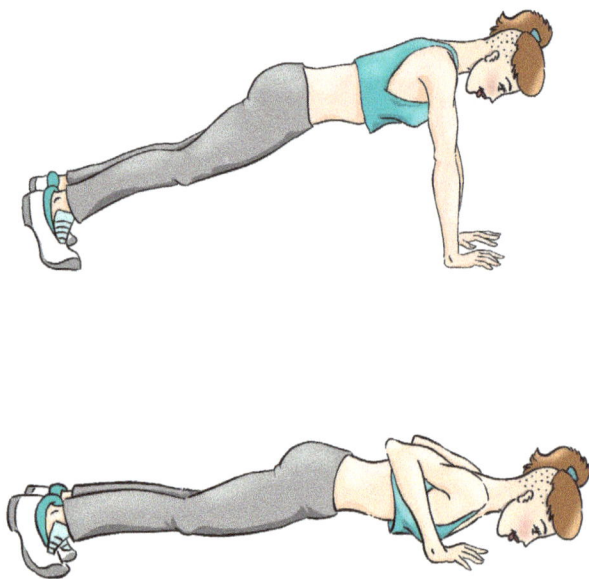

Beginner Level 1:

The push-up can be performed on your knees and using a chair/table/bench. While on your knees, keep your body straight and your core activated and place your hands on the edge of your chosen piece of furniture. Lower your chest until it touches the edge of the furniture and forcefully push your body back up to the starting position, keeping your body as straight as possible.

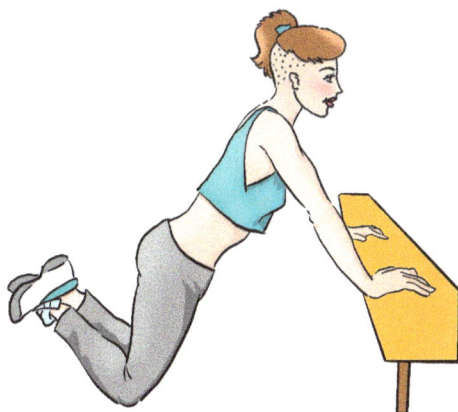

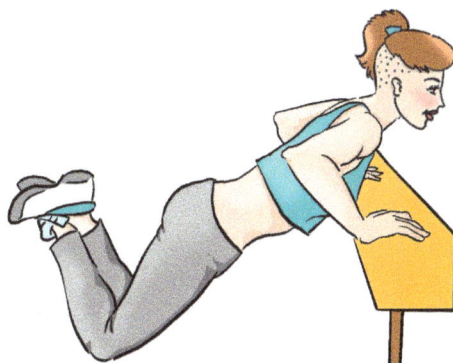

Beginner level 2:

The push-up can also be performed on your knees, without the chair/table/bench. As above, stay on your knees and lower your chest to a floor/mat/towel rather than a bench. Keeping your body straight, push back up to the starting position.

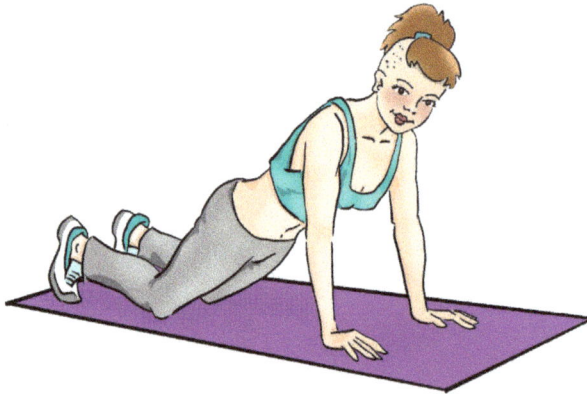

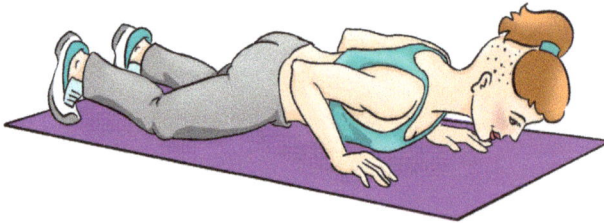

Inchworm

This is a variation of a plank that is excellent for strengthening the shoulders and core.

Stand completely erect. Keeping your back straight, bend forward, hinging at your hips to bring your hands to the floor and bending your knees if you feel too much pressure on your hamstrings (the back of your legs). Walk your hands forward, moving into a high plank/top of a push-up position. Now walk your hands back towards your feet, keeping your core activated (abs and glutes tight) and your back as straight as possible, and return to a standing position. This is one repetition.

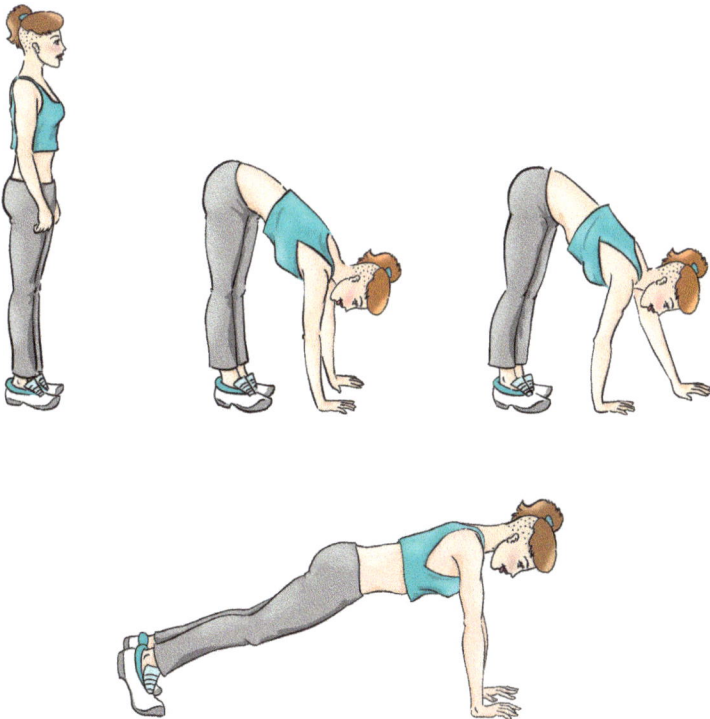

High plank

The plank is one of the best isometric strength exercises that you can do for your core. (Isometric strength − or static strength − exercises involve holding a position for a certain period of time rather than moving.) Depending on the plank you perform, you will also build strength in your shoulders, arms, glutes and legs.

Start by lying down as if you were about to do a push up. Place your palms on the floor next to your shoulders and flex your feet, with your toes and the balls of your feet pressed down on the floor. Take a deep breath and raise yourself into a push-up position. Holding the top of your push-up, your body should be in a straight line, from your heels to the top of your head. Draw your naval/belly button in towards your spine and squeeze your glutes/buttocks. Ensure your shoulders and shoulder blades are pulled down away from your neck and ears, lengthening through your spine. Look at the floor to keep your head and neck in a neutral position. Try not to hold your breath and instead breathe normally.

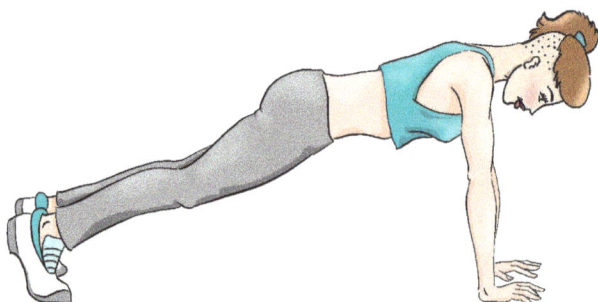

Plank on forearms/elbows

This is the most popular way to perform the plank position.

Rest your forearms on the ground, with your elbows aligned directly below your shoulders. If placing your palms on the floor feels uncomfortable, clasp your hands together. As with the high plank, as you raise yourself up, ensure your body is in a straight line and keep your core activated.

This form of the plank position can also be performed while resting on your knees (see second illustration). Again, just make sure your body is in a straight line and your core is activated.

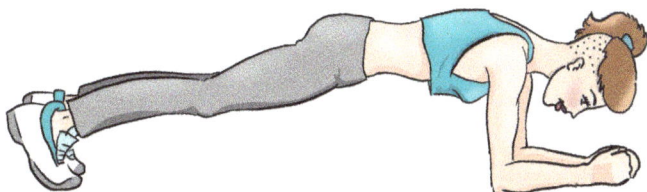

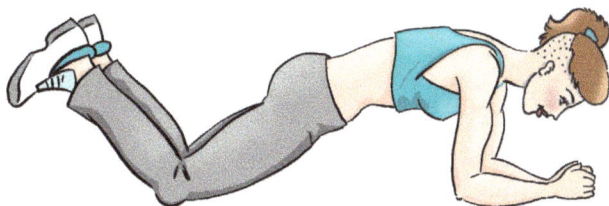

Plank shoulder tap

This variation of the plank position is a more challenging movement; its focus is on core stability rather than excessive movement.

Begin in the high plank position (the hands and feet position for the more advanced and the hands and knee position for beginners). Ensure your hands are directly under your shoulders, with your feet or knees slightly wider apart to provide a stable base. It is important to remain as stable as possible during this movement. To avoid unnecessary stress on your shoulders and lower back, brace your abs, squeeze your glutes and pull in your naval towards your spine. Maintain a straight line with your body and then lift one hand off the ground, moving it in a controlled manner to touch the opposite shoulder. Keep your hips square to the ground and avoid rotating your body as you lift your hand. Try to maintain a straight line and don't let your hips rise or fall. Alternate the movement between the left and right.

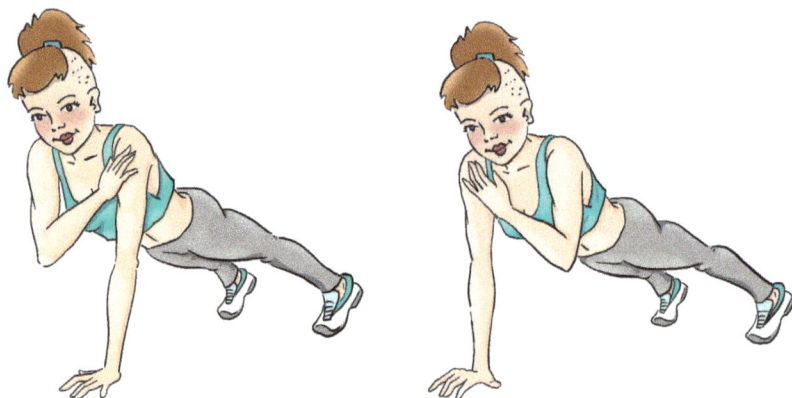

Plank toe tap

This movement will help tone and strengthen your shoulders, lower back and glutes.

Start in the basic plank position and alternate between moving each leg one to two feet to the side, tap the floor and then return to the start position. While doing this exercise, keep your glutes squeezed, your abdominals tight and your naval drawn inwards. Try not to let your hips rise or fall and keep the movement slow and controlled.

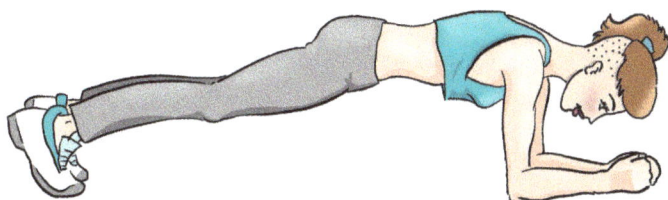

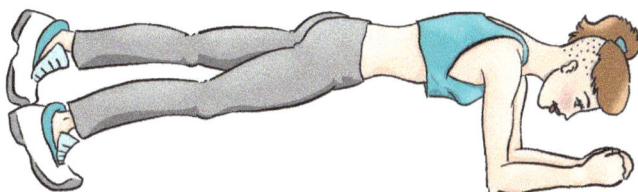

Dip

The triceps dip is a great body weight exercise that builds arm and shoulder strength. Core activation (keeping your abdominal muscles tight) is required during this movement.

Start by sitting on the edge of a chair with your hands clasping the end of the seat next to your hips. With your fingers pointing forward, your legs extended, your feet approximately hip-width apart and your heels down, press into your palms to lift your body off the chair and slide forward just enough so that your buttocks clear the edge of the seat. Now lower yourself until your elbows are bent at approximately a 45-degree angle and then slowly push yourself back up to the starting position. This is one repetition. Avoid locking your elbows or allowing your hips to shift forwards, away from the chair.

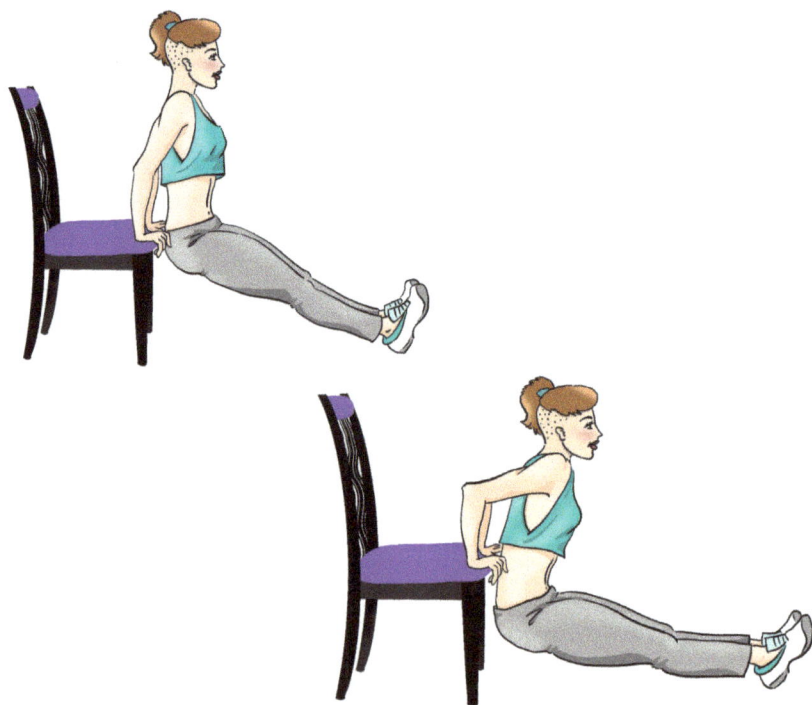

If keeping your legs fully extended feels too hard, you can bend your knees, keeping them perpendicular (at 90 degrees) to the ground. This reduces your body weight, therefore making the dip slightly easier.

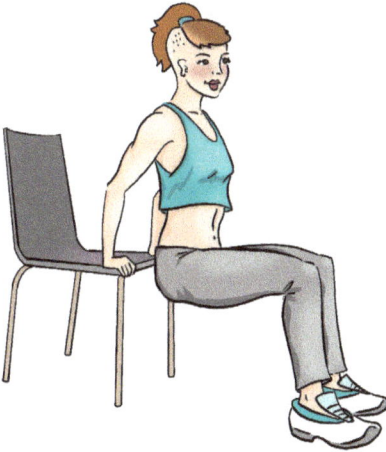

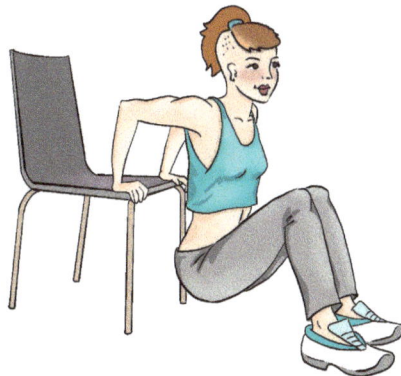

Mountain climber

This bodyweight exercise is useful for burning calories, building stamina and strengthening your shoulders and core.

Start the movement in a high plank position. Ensure that your hands are directly under your shoulders and maintain a tight core (squeeze your buttocks and keep your abdominal muscles active by imagining that you are pulling your belly button to the back of your spine). Keeping this position, pull one knee up and inwards towards your midsection. This movement should be as smooth and as controlled as possible, so try not to let your body rise up or sag down. Extend the leg back to the starting position and repeat with the other leg. Each high knee/leg movement is counted as one repetition.

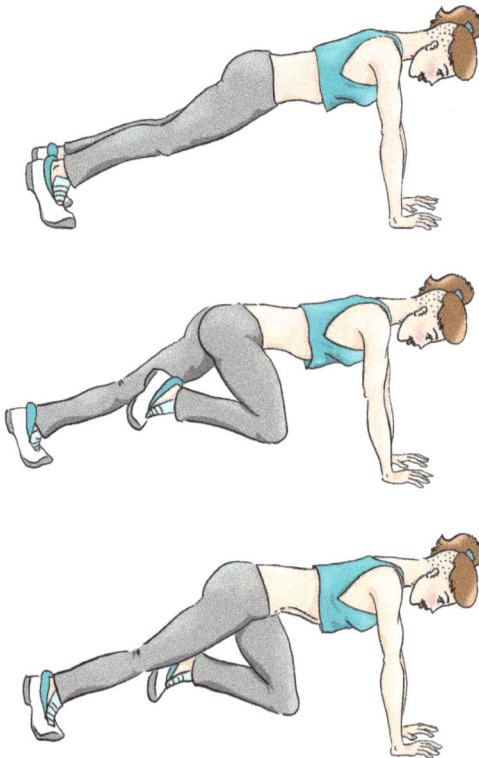

Bear crawl

A bear crawl is a bodyweight mobility movement. It is a functional exercise that helps build strength in your shoulders, quads (front of the thighs) and abdominal muscles.

Start the movement on all fours on the floor. Lift your knees, so that your legs form a 90-degree angle with the floor, with your knees just hovering an inch or so above it. Keep your back straight, your core strong and engaged (you will feel your abdominals tense and activated in this position), your legs hip-width apart and your arms shoulder-width apart. Now move one hand and the opposite foot forward and then proceed with the opposite side, as if crawling like a bear. Concentrate on keeping your knees low to the ground, which will focus the movement on the core area (back and abdominals). Avoid shrugging your shoulders by keeping your shoulders and scapula drawn downwards.

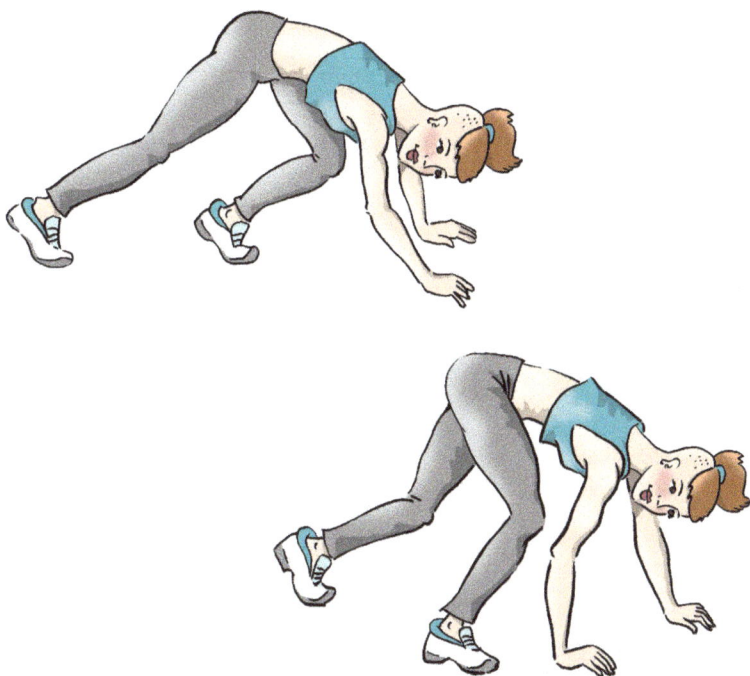

Crab walk

If you're new to it, this will seem like a rather strange bodyweight movement, but that aside, it will ensure a full body workout.

Start by sitting on the floor with your feet out in front of you, hip-width apart. Place your hands, palms down, on the floor behind your hips and slightly to the side of them. Now push up onto your hands and feet, raising your hips as high off the ground as possible. Start by moving one hand and the opposite foot forward, alternating between left and right, thus inching forward on all fours. During the movement, concentrate on keeping your hips high.

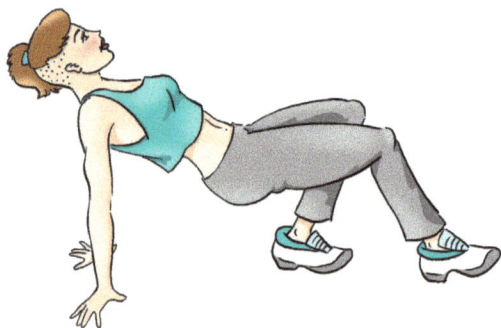

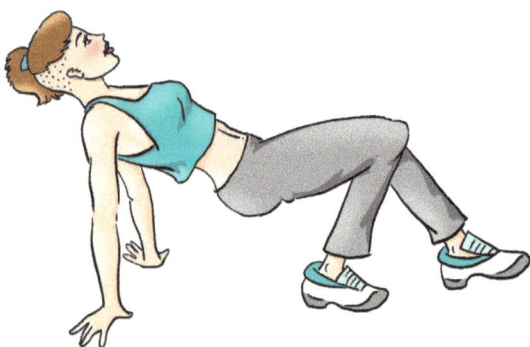

Lower Body

Squat

The bodyweight squat is a lower body strengthening exercise that can be performed virtually anywhere, with no equipment and in limited space. It is a highly functional movement that works all the major muscles in your legs.

Start with your feet shoulder-width apart and your toes slightly out, your heels flat. Keep your core tight (abdominal muscles engaged) and hinge at the hips, bending your knees so that your hips move towards the ground (just as you would sit in a chair). Pause for a moment at the bottom of the squat and then push back up to a standing position, with your knees pushing outwards. To counterbalance your weight, hold your arms out in front of you at shoulder height. Aim to keep your back straight/flat during the entire movement.

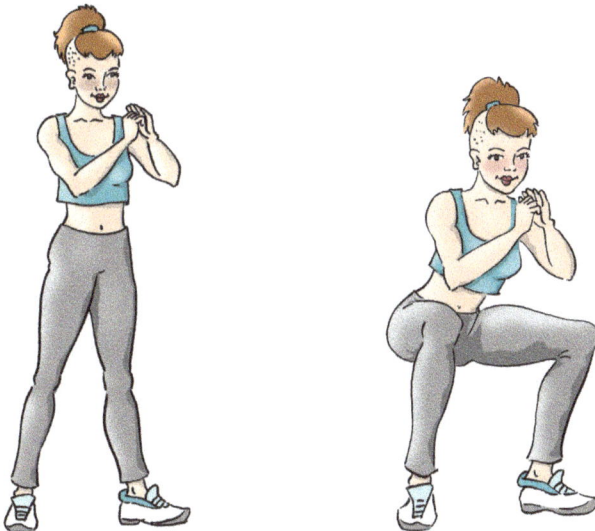

Lunge

A lunge is a single-leg bodyweight exercise that works your hips, glutes, quads, hamstrings, core and inner thigh muscles. It helps to develop lower body strength and endurance.

Stand with your feet hip-width apart, keeping your back straight, your shoulders back and your abdominal muscles tight. Take a step forward, bending both knees and lowering your back one until it touches the floor. At this point, your front leg should be at a 90-degree angle to the floor. Return to the standing position by pushing up through your front foot. This is one repetition. Alternate the movement, repeating with your alternate leg touching the floor.

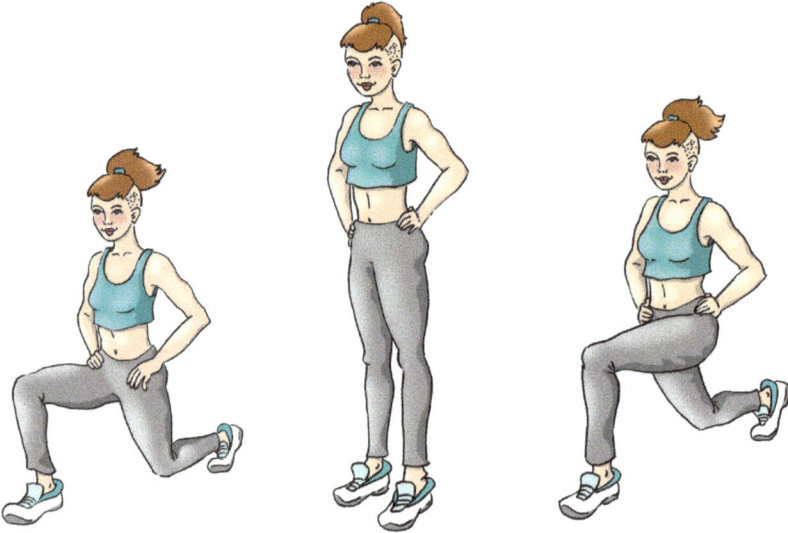

Side lunge

Side lunges work your glutes, quads and hamstrings, and they have the added bonus of tackling both your outer and inner thighs.

Initiate the movement by standing with your feet hip-width apart. Step out to the side with your left leg, bend your left knee and push your hips back. Aim to get your hips and buttocks as low to the ground as possible, keeping your back flat and straight, your core engaged, and your abs squeezed tight. Push back to the starting position and repeat the movement with your right leg. If you need to, use your arms for balance by extending them forward at shoulder height.

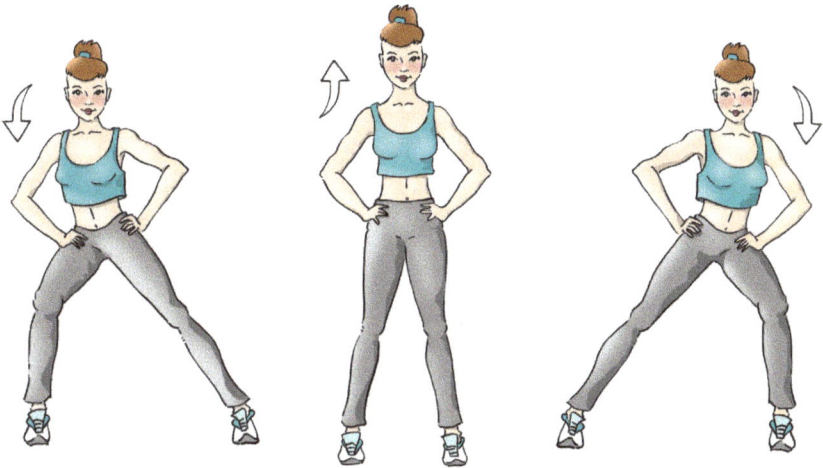

Good morning

Good mornings provide an excellent workout for the hamstrings, glutes and lower back (the posterior chain).

Stand with your feet shoulder-width apart and your hands behind your head. Stand upright, brace your core and pull your shoulders back. Take a breath and hinge forward from your hips (not from your waist), allowing a slight bend in your knees. Keeping your back flat, bend forward until you feel a slight pull in your hamstrings (do not bend beyond a 90-degree angle). Then, as you exhale, reverse the movement to stand up straight. Keep your core engaged throughout the entire movement and really focus on squeezing your glutes (buttocks) as you stand up.

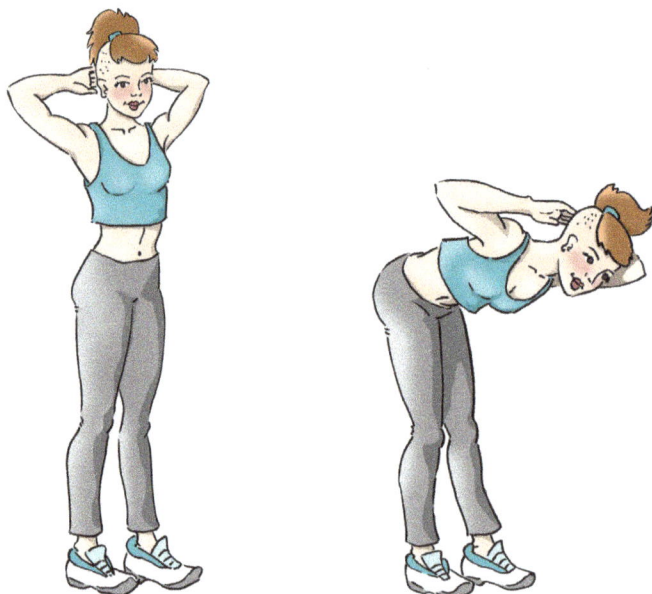

Sumo squat

These focus mainly on the glutes and the inner thighs, but the muscles that will benefit are the quads, hamstrings, upper flexors and calves.

Stand with your feet in a wide stance and your toes pointing out to the side. When doing the sumo squat, keep your back flat and your abdominal muscles (core) engaged. Lower yourself by bending your knees and pushing your hips back, ensuring that your knees stay in line with your toes. When your thighs are parallel to the floor, return to the starting position. This is one repetition completed.

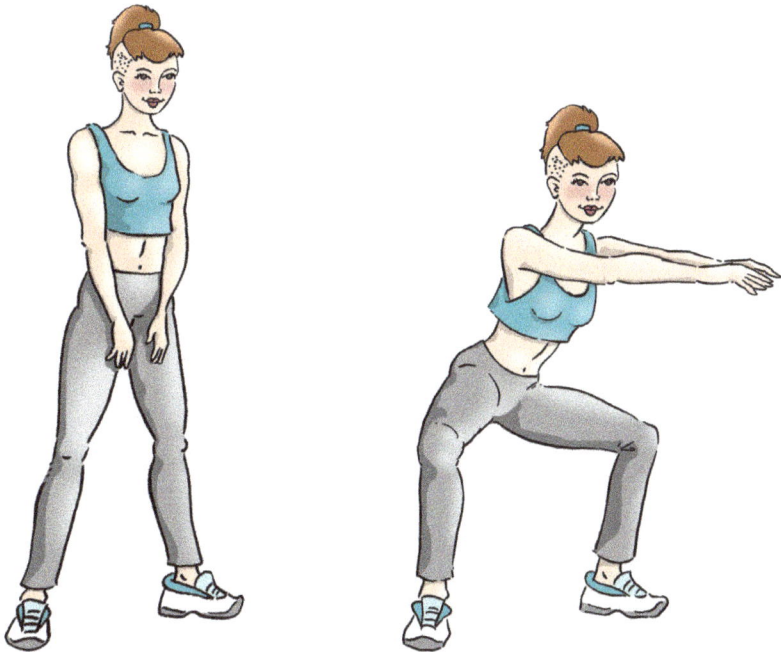

Glute bridge

As the name suggests, this exercise will help to strengthen your glutes (buttocks), core and hamstrings.

Start the movement by lying on your back with your hands by your side, your knees bent and your feet flat on the ground. Lift your hips off the floor whilst keeping your back straight and your abdominal muscles tight, pushing your hips up as high as possible. Squeeze your glutes at the top of the movement and hold for three seconds, before slowly lowering your hips back to the floor whilst keeping control of your movement and pace. That is one repetition completed. Focus on keeping your core and glutes engaged throughout the movement.

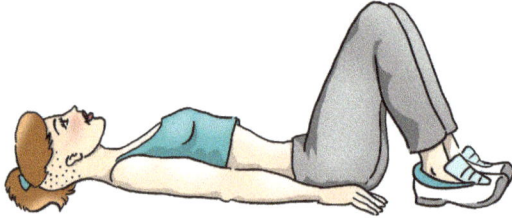

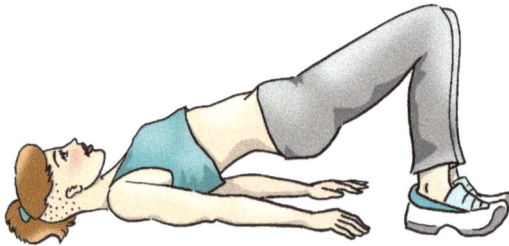

LOWER BODY

Bulgarian split squat

This is a great exercise for improving your balance and knee stability, and for strengthening your posterior chain of muscles (glutes and hamstrings). It's also extremely beneficial for runners. You will need a step, an exercise box or a sturdy chair.

Stand up tall in front of the step, box or chair, then bend your knee and rest your right foot on top of it. Keep your back straight and your core engaged and bend your left knee, lowering your right one as far as possible to the ground. Push forcefully through your heel and return to a standing position. This is one repetition. Now place your left toes on the step, box or chair and repeat the movement with your right leg.

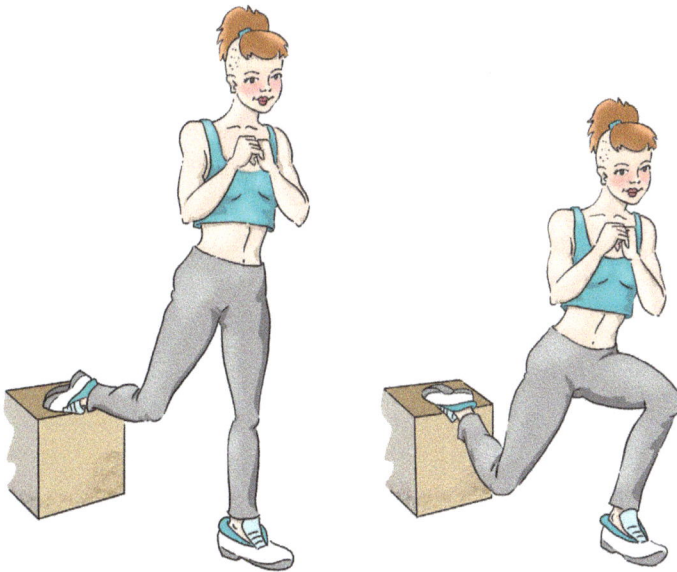

Fire hydrant

Fire hydrants target the outer glutes, core and hips.

Start the movement on all fours on your exercise mat or towel, ensuring your wrists are directly under your shoulders, your knees are hip-width apart and your toes are flexed on the ground (hips, knees and ankles should all be at 90-degree angles to the floor).

Keeping your knee bent, raise your left leg out to the side until your knee is level with your hip and return to the starting position. This is one repetition.

When performing this movement, ensure you keep your neck neutral by looking down at the floor and avoid arching your back by engaging your core. Focus on keeping your elbows locked and your weight centralised. There should be no leaning over to the support side.

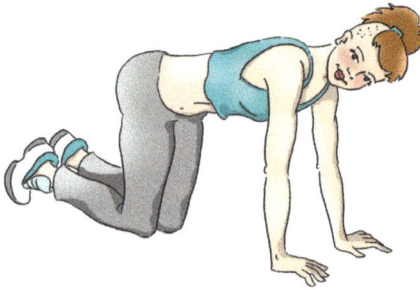

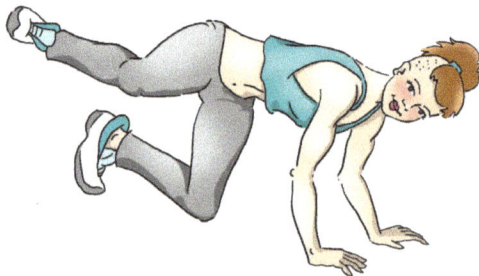

Bird dog

This is a great exercise to add to your workout, as it will strengthen your core and improve your balance and overall posture. I highly recommend it for anyone who suffers from lower back pain, as it will help to improve the stability of the lumber spine.

Start the movement on all fours, with your hands directly under your shoulders and your knees under your hips and hip-width apart. Simultaneously extend your left leg backward and your right arm forward. Hold for a count of three seconds and return to the start position. This is one repetition. Switch sides and repeat, extending your right leg to the rear while stretching out your left arm.

Keep your neck in a neutral position by looking down at the floor throughout the movement. In addition, engage your core and avoid arching your back.

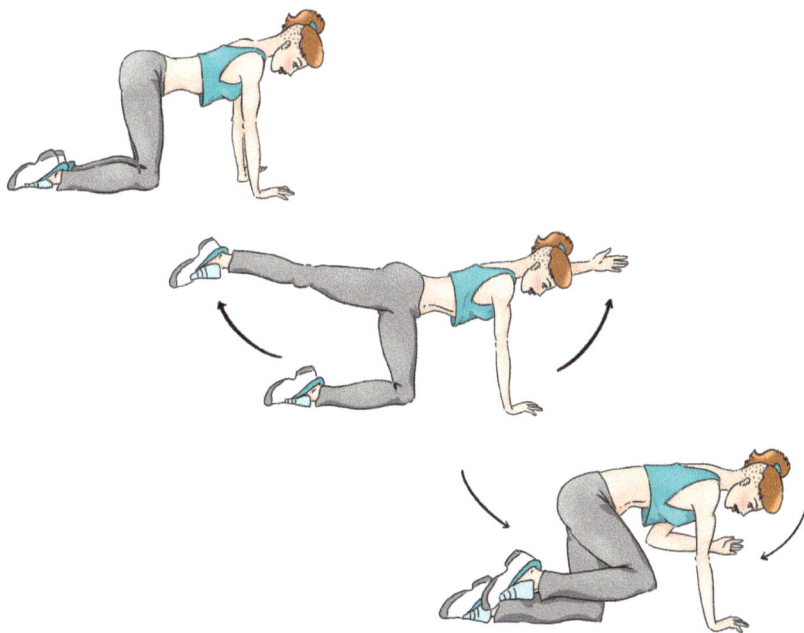

Bear crawl

A bear crawl is a bodyweight mobility movement. It is a functional exercise that helps build strength in your shoulders, quads (front of the thighs) and abdominal muscles.

Start the movement on all fours on the floor. Lift your knees, so that your legs form a 90-degree angle with the floor, with your knees hovering an inch or so above it. Keep your back straight and your core strong and engaged (you will feel your abdominals tense and activated in this position). Your legs should be hip-width apart and your arms shoulder-width apart. Now move one hand and the opposite foot forward, before switching to the opposite side, as if crawling like a bear. Concentrate on keeping your knees low to the ground, as this will focus the movement on the core area (back and abdominals). Avoid shrugging your shoulders by keeping them pointing downwards.

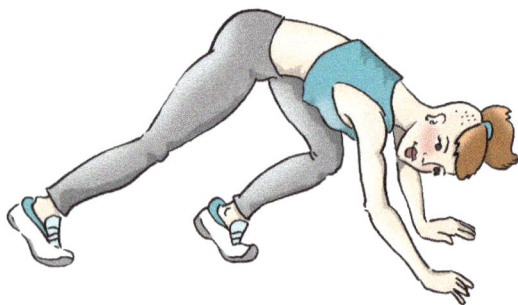

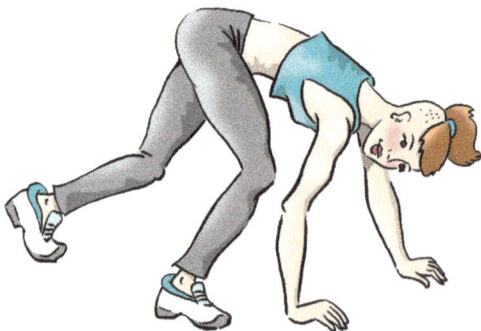

Curtsy lunge

The curtsy lunge is a variation on the traditional lunge that targets the inner thighs, as well as the gluteal medius muscle of the buttock. It will also engage the quads, hamstrings, calves and back.

Start the movement by standing tall with your feet wider than shoulder-width apart and your hands on your hips. Step your left leg behind and to the right, so that your thighs cross, bending both knees as if you are curtsying. Push back up to the start position and switch to the other leg. During this movement, focus on keeping your core (abdominal muscles) engaged and your back straight.

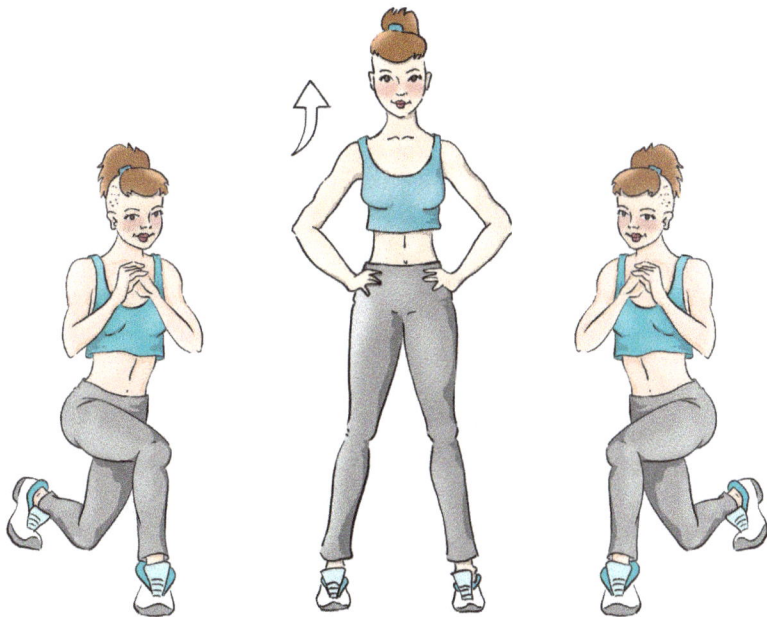

Reverse lunge high knee

This is a great exercise, as it targets most of the leg muscles. It also improves balance and is, therefore, a great exercise for runners.

Start by standing tall, with your feet hip-width apart. Step back with your right leg and bend both knees until they make a 90-degree angle. Stand back up and, as you do so, bring your right knee forward and up until it reaches your chest. Now for the challenging part. Without putting your right foot on the ground, bring it back for the next repetition, thus going straight into the next lunge. Ensure you keep your core and glutes engaged. During this movement, you can also use your arms to stabilise and control your balance.

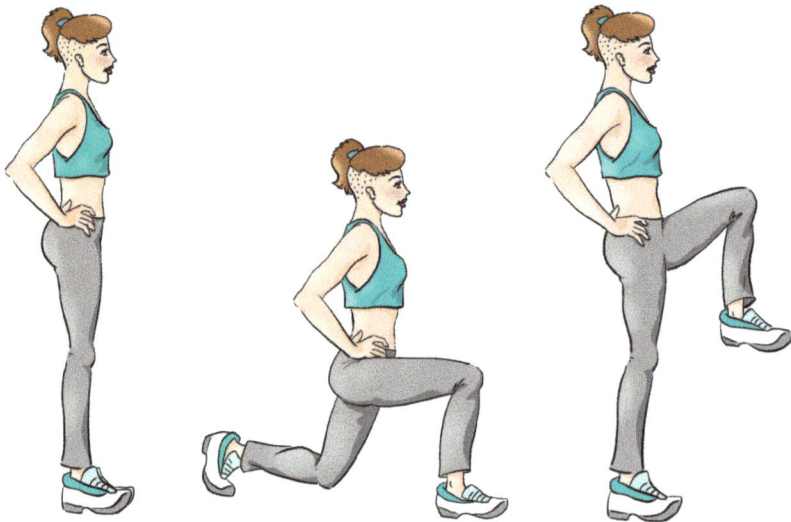

Metabolic Conditioning Exercises

Burpee

Burpees increase the heart rate and build strength and stamina, providing an intense metabolic conditioning workout that uses all the major muscle groups and burns multiple calories in a short space of time. They also increase agility and flexibility.

Begin in an upright position, with your feet shoulder-width apart. Bend forward and place both hands on the ground in front of your feet. Jump or step back until both legs are fully extended behind your body and you are in the high plank position. Lower your body to the ground (lying prone on the floor). Push your chest back up until you are in a high plank position again and jump or step your feet forward towards your hands, before moving into a standing position. This is one repetition completed. Avoid arching your back when lowering yourself down to the floor, especially when fatigued, by squeezing your glutes and abdominal muscles.

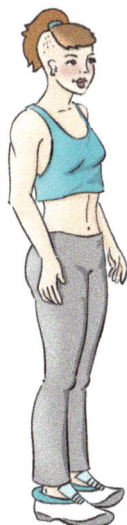

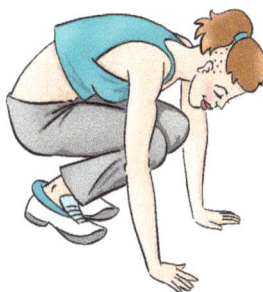

Burpee continued

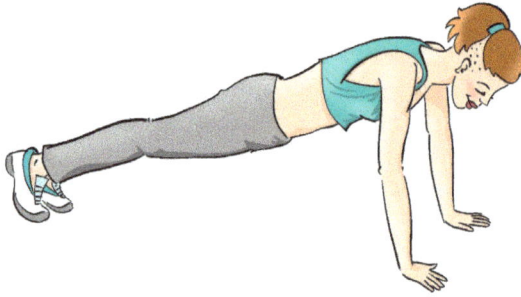

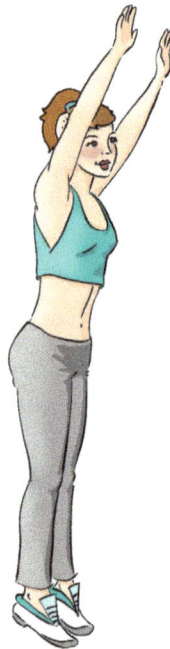

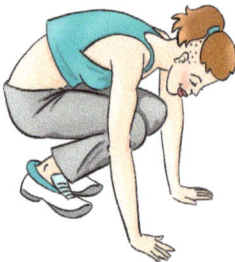

Jumping jack

Jumping jacks provide a great full body workout, and they increase muscle endurance and cardiovascular capacity.

Start the movement by standing completely upright, with your feet together and your hands at your sides. Jump up and out with your feet, and at the same time bring both of your hands together above your head. Jump up and in with your feet and return your arms to your sides. When jumping, keep your knees slightly bent and land softly on the balls of your feet. During the exercise, try and maintain a steady and smooth rhythm and control your breathing with regular, deep breaths.

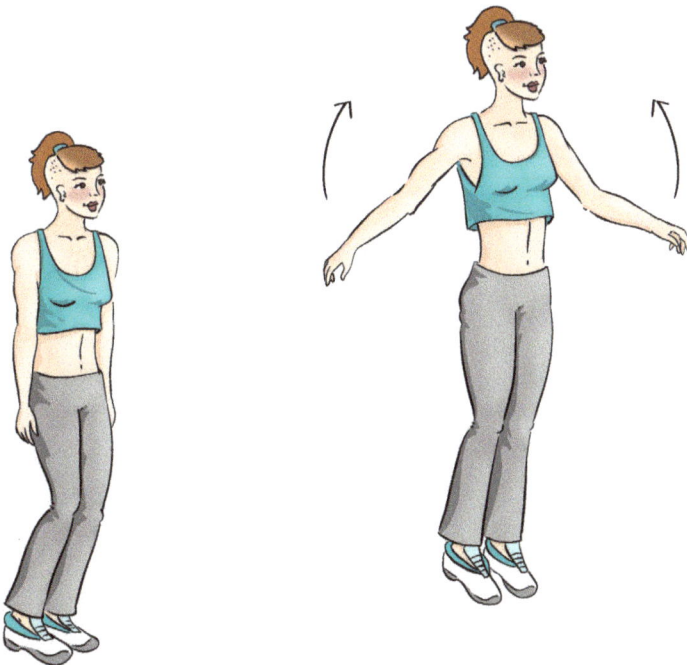

Jumping jack continued

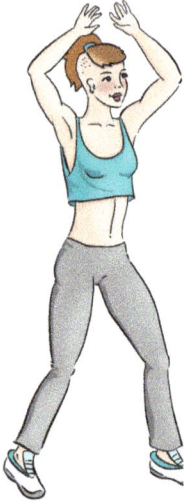

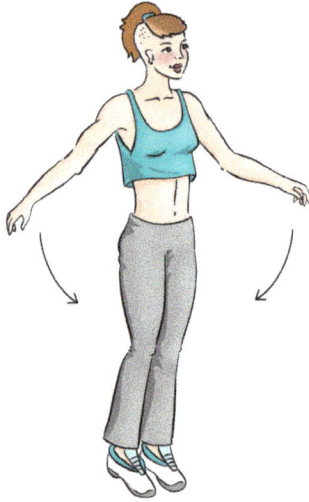

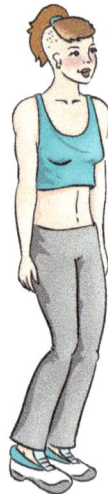

High knee

This cardiovascular exercise is designed to be performed at a fast pace and will engage your core, strengthen all the muscles in your legs and elevate your heart rate in a very short space of time. This means it's great for a full body warm up.

Stand upright with your feet shoulder-width apart. Face forwards with your core engaged and your chest up and open. Bring your knees up to waist height or as high as possible (one at a time) and then slowly land on the balls of your feet. Once you have practised this movement a few times, you can start to speed it up. Ensure that your shoulders are back and your arms are swinging in a controlled movement (similar to that of a sprinter). Keep your impact with the ground light and focused and control your breathing.

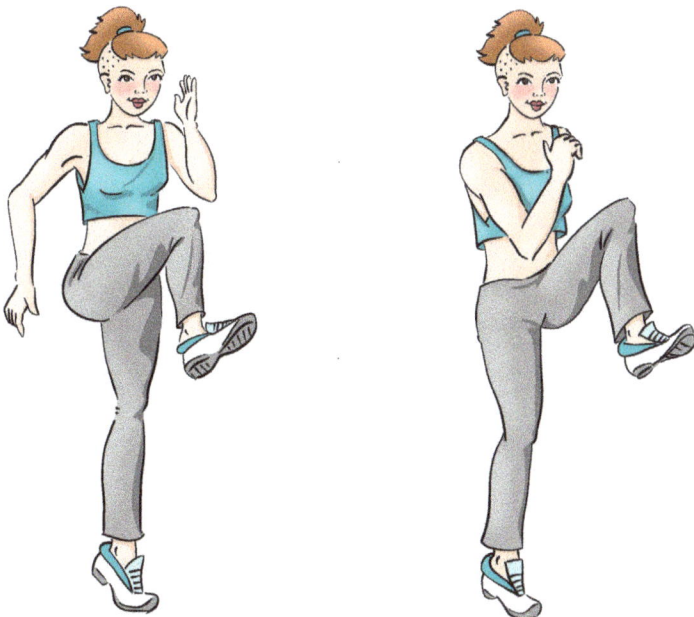

Heel flick

This is a great metabolic conditioning movement. It is often used as a warm-up exercise, but for a bit of a cardio hit it can be incorporated into any workout.

Stand tall with your feet shoulder-width apart and your core engaged.

Start by kicking your heels up towards your glutes. Try to touch your heel to them, while at the same time pumping your arms at your sides, as if you were sprinting. Remember to keep your chest up and your shoulders back, and land softly on the balls of your feet.

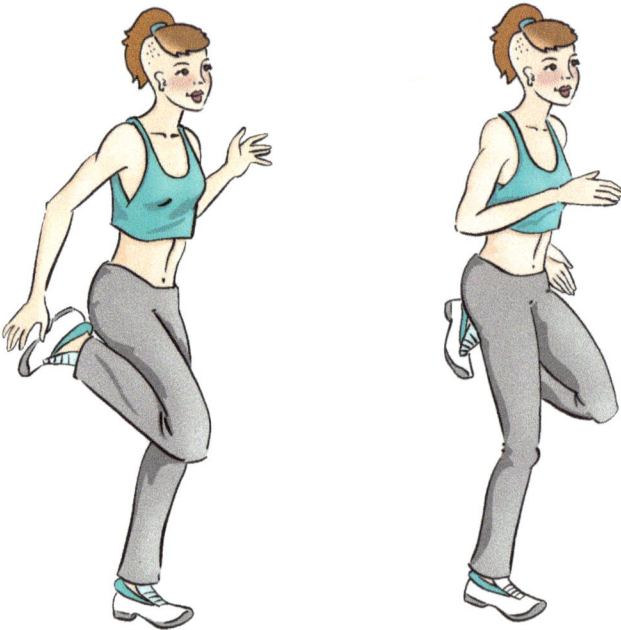

In-and-out running on the spot

This exercise is great for building speed and agility. It will also increase your heart rate for a great cardio workout.

Stand in an athletic position with your feet shoulder-width apart and your hips flexed and low. Stay on the balls of your feet. Pushing through them, run on the spot as fast as possible (tap-tap-tap), while moving ever so slightly in-and-out laterally (sideways) with your feet. Stay low throughout the movement and use your arms for support and balance. Keep your core engaged and stay light on your feet. Try to focus on a steady, even breathing pattern (deep breaths).

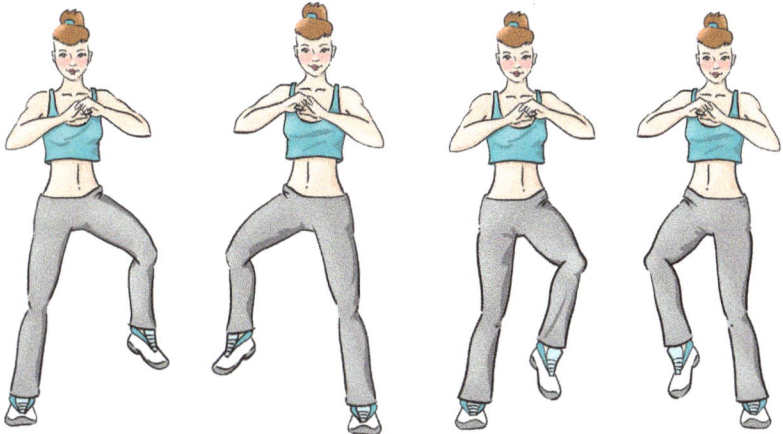

Mountain climber

Mountain climbers are a dynamic, whole body movement, which, when performed at a quick pace, will increase your overall aerobic fitness, flexibility and agility.

Start with your body in the high plank position, with your hands slightly wider than your shoulders, your core engaged and your back as straight as possible. Now bring one knee up to your belly button, swap legs and do the same.

Begin at a moderate pace and when you are comfortable with the exercise, increase the speed of your knee movement, which will intensify the impact of the cardio workout. When you feel yourself getting tired, concentrate on keeping your core engaged and your back straight.

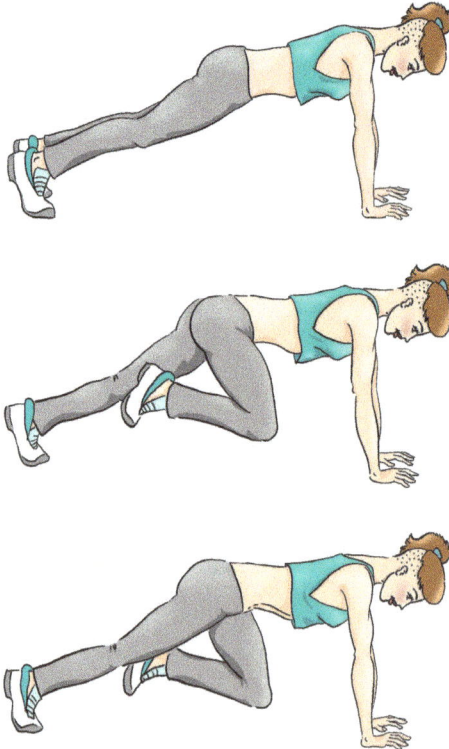

Squat hop

This movement is great for building leg and gluteal strength and endurance. As it is a plyometric movement (also known as jump training or plyos, these are exercises in which the muscles exert the maximum effort over short intervals, with the goal of increasing their power), it will also stimulate your cardiovascular system.

Stand with your feet apart, slightly wider than your hips. Lower your body into a squat position. Press up through your feet, engage your abdominals and jump up explosively, lifting your arms up as you do so. Upon landing, lower yourself back down into a squat position, ready for the next jump.

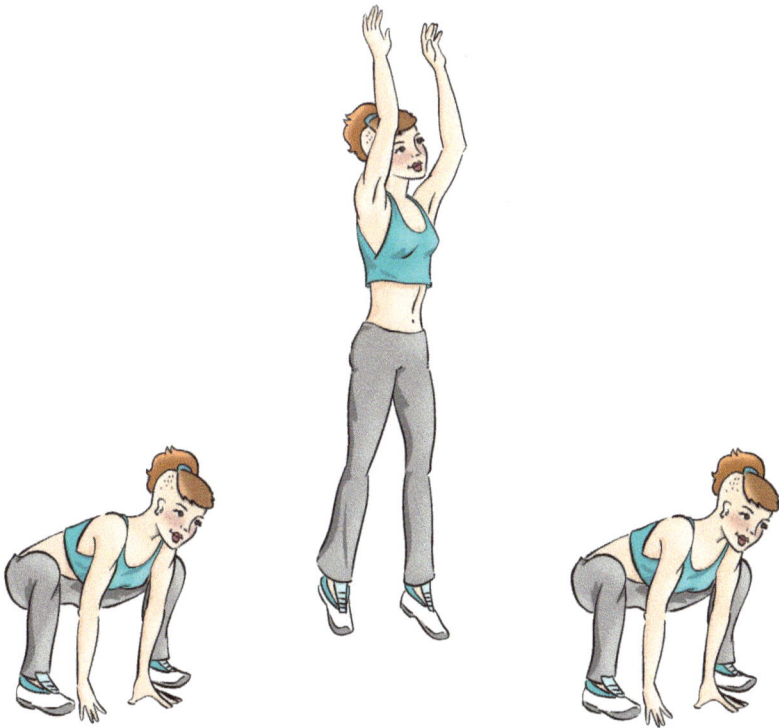

Bear crawl

A bear crawl is a bodyweight mobility movement. It is a functional exercise that helps build strength in your shoulders, quads (front of the thighs) and abdominal muscles.

Start the movement on all fours on the floor. Lift your knees, so that your legs form a 90-degree angle with the floor, your knees just hovering an inch or so above it. Keep your back straight, your core strong and engaged (you will feel your abdominals tense and activated in this position) your legs hip-width apart and your arms shoulder-width apart. Now move one hand and the opposite foot forward and then proceed with the opposite side, as if crawling forwards like a bear. Concentrate on keeping your knees low to the ground, which will focus the movement on the core area (back and abdominals). Avoid shrugging your shoulders by keeping your shoulders and scapula drawn downwards.

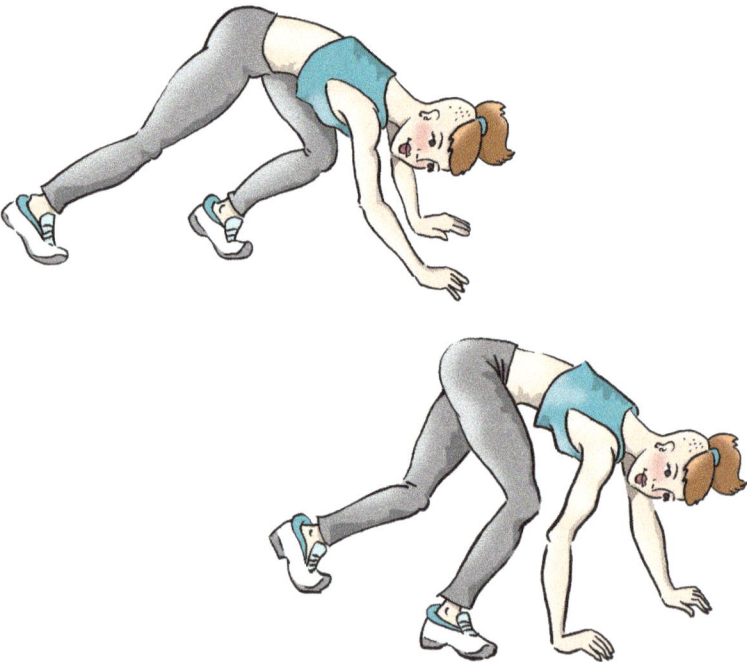

Crab walk

If you're new to it, this will seem like a rather strange bodyweight movement, but that aside, it will ensure a full body workout.

Start by sitting on the floor with your feet out in front of you, hip-width apart. Place your hands, palms down, on the floor behind your hips and slightly to the side of them. Now push up onto your hands and feet, raising your hips as high off the ground as possible. Start by moving one hand and the opposite foot forward, alternating between left and right, thus inching forward on all fours. During the movement, concentrate on keeping your hips high.

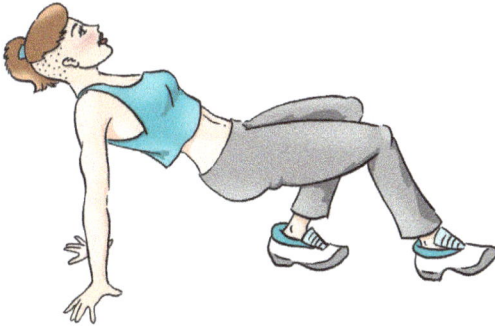

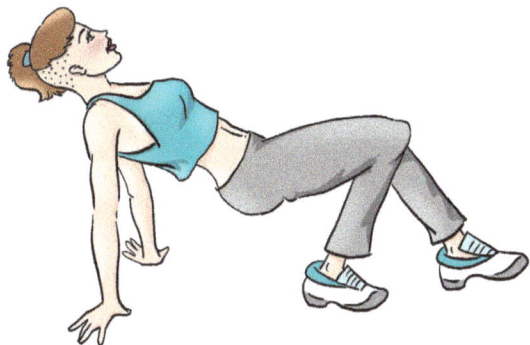

Skater

This is a great cardiovascular movement, which will also help with agility and balance.

Begin in an athletic standing position. (In other words, stand in a quarter squat, with your feet flat and wider than your hips and your back straight. This is also known as the 'ready position'.) Lean forward, and with your right foot jump to the right, bringing your left foot up behind you. Use your arms for balance and power in an exaggerated sprinting motion. From this position, jump to the left, incorporating your arms in just the same way. These two movements should replicate a speed skater gliding across the ice.

Focus on keeping your core engaged and your back flat. Land lightly on the balls of your feet.

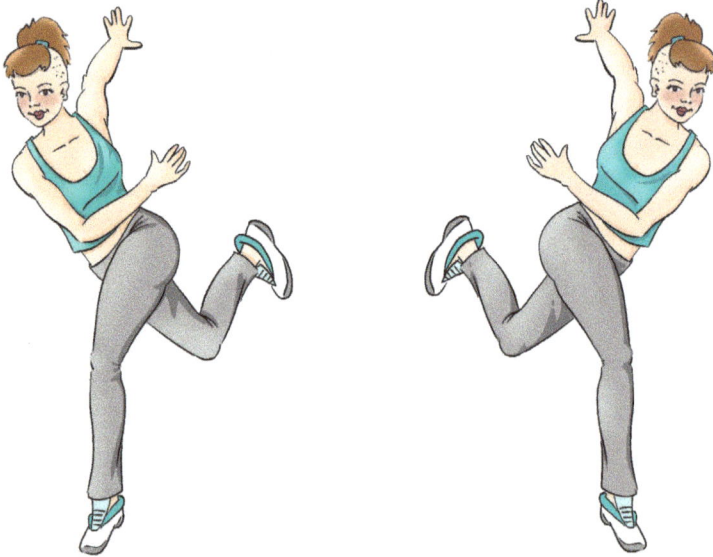

Side hop

A side hop is mainly a plyometric exercise (also known as jump training or plyos, these are exercises in which the muscles exert the maximum effort over short intervals, with the goal of increasing their power), which will tax your cardiovascular system. It is fantastic for agility, speed and explosiveness.

Start the movement by standing tall, with your hands at your sides and your feet hip-width apart. Jump with both feet to the right and then as quickly as possible to the left. Repeat this movement from right to left.

Try not to lock your knees and focus on landing softly on the balls of your feet. Keep your core engaged and concentrate on controlling your breath during the jumps.

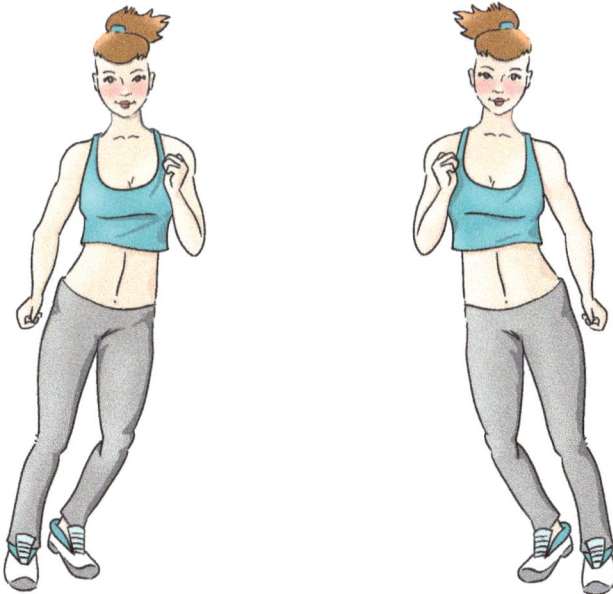

METABOLIC CONDITIONING

Frog hop

Frog hops are another great plyometric exercise, and they will add some variety and spice to your workout routine.

Start the movement in a squat position, with your knees and toes pointing outwards, your back straight and your core engaged. Jump up and forward, landing as smoothly as possible back into the squat position. This is one repetition completed.

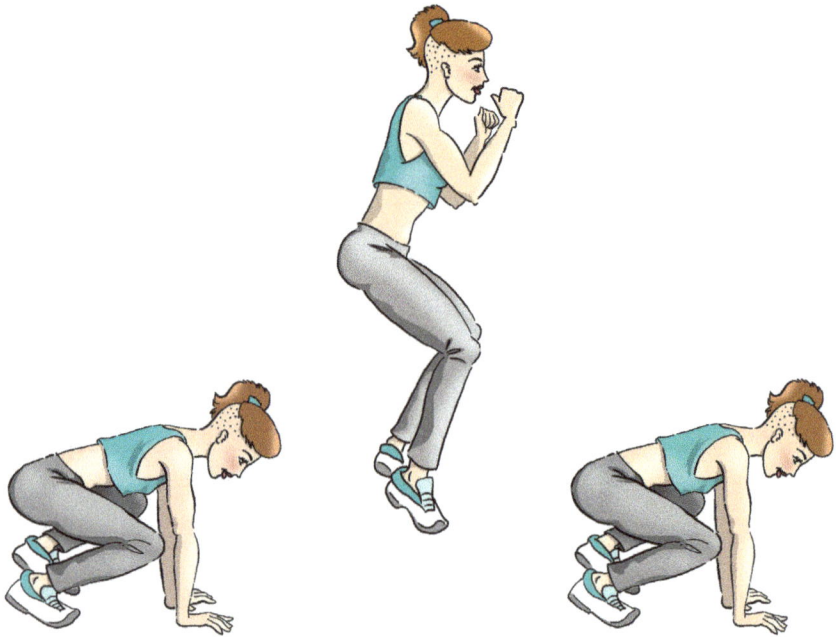

Core, Abdominals and Back

Sit-up

Sit-ups might seem easy, but when they are performed correctly and in a controlled manner, they are a great movement to strengthen the abdominal muscles.

Start by lying on your back on your mat or a towel. Bend your knees and place the soles of your feet against each other (butterfly/flop your knees outwards). By doing butterfly sit-ups, you will prevent the hip flexor muscles from doing the majority of the work. Now lift your torso/upper body into a sitting position and then lower yourself until you are lying down again. This is one repetition completed. During the sit-ups, focus on using your abdominals to perform the majority of the movement, although it's OK if you find yourself using your arms for a bit of momentum.

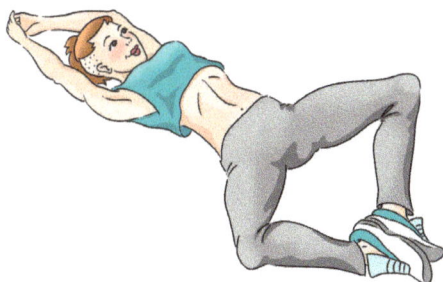

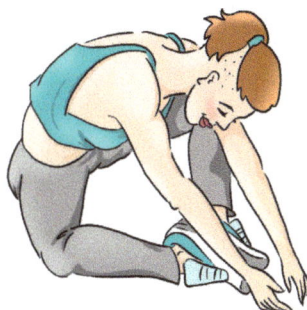

Crunch

Crunches target the upper abdominals (the area just below the sternum). By strengthening your abdominal muscles, you also strengthen your core. A strong core is important for stability, balance and good posture.

Start by lying down on your mat or towel, with your knees bent, your back and feet flat on the ground and your fingers lightly touching the sides of your head (your temples). Now raise your shoulders and the top of your chest from the ground, squeeze your upper abdominals (you should feel tension just below your sternum) and then slowly lower yourself to the starting position. This is one repetition completed. When doing crunches, do not interlace your fingers behind your head. This is because as you get tired, it will become tempting to pull on the back of your head, which can lead to injury or pain in the neck.

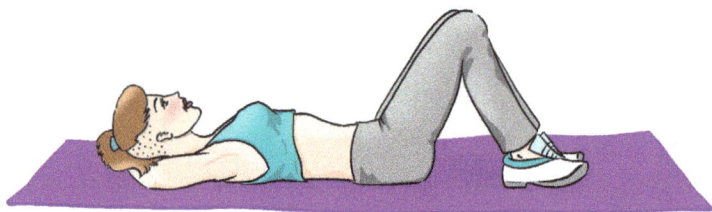

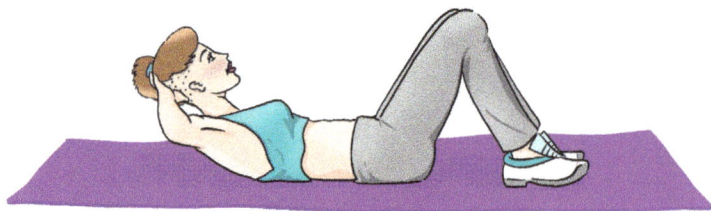

Leg raise

The leg raise is an abdominal and anterior hip flexor strengthening exercise.

Lie supine (facing up) on your mat or towel. Place your hands under your lower back for support, while keeping it in contact with the ground. Try and keep your legs as straight as possible. (If you feel too much tension in your hamstrings – the back of your legs – you can bend them slightly.) Lift your legs up in a controlled manner until they are at a 90-degree angle with the ground. Now slowly lower your legs back down (do not slam or drop them) and gently touch your heels to your mat. This is one repetition completed. During the movement, focus on pressing your lower back into your mat, with your abdominal muscles engaged.

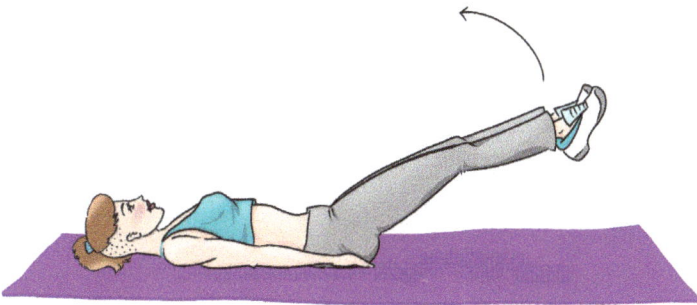

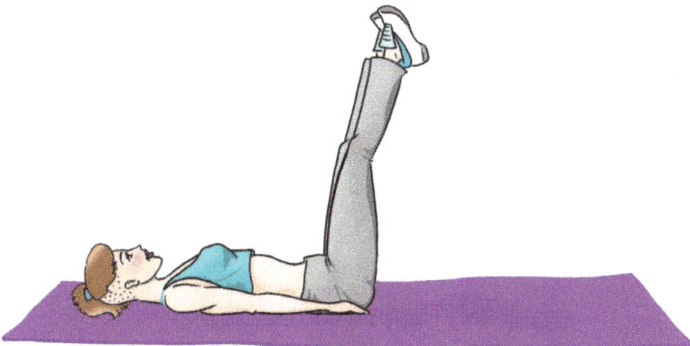

Single leg raise

This is a slightly easier version of the leg raise.

Start by lying supine on your mat or towel. Keep your left leg straight and your right leg bent, with the sole of your right foot flat on the ground. Place your hands under your lower back, keeping it in contact with your mat. Lift your left leg up until it is at a 90-degree angle to the ground and then slowly lower it back down to your mat. This is one repetition completed. Carry out a number of repetitions with your left leg, before switching to your right one. Keep your movements slow and controlled and remember to keep your lower back in constant contact with your mat.

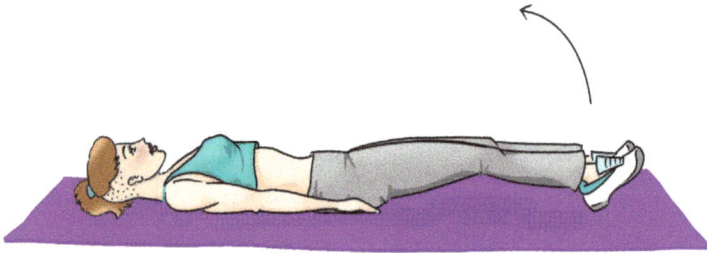

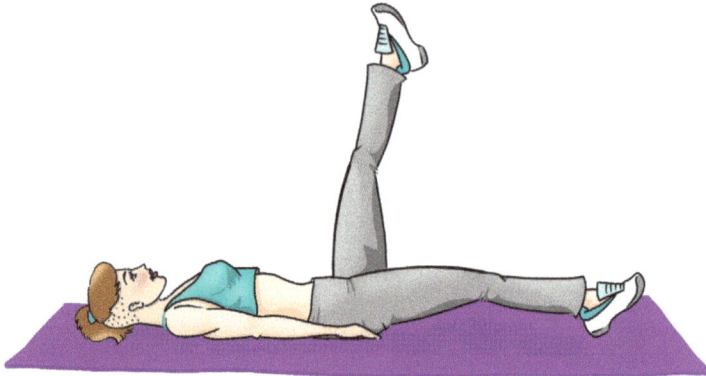

Bicycle

Bicycles are a challenging but highly effective core strengthening exercise.

Start by lying on your mat or towel, with your lower back pressing down and in contact with the ground. Raise your shoulders and head slightly off the ground, with your hands at your temples (don't interlace your fingers behind your head). Lift one leg off the ground and extend it out, now lift your other and bend your knee towards your chest. As you do this, twist through your core so the opposite arm/elbow comes towards the raised/bent knee.

Focus on moving through your core as you turn your torso/chest. Do not pull on your head or think of it as a shoulder-to-knee action rather than an elbow-to-knee one. Now alternate to the opposite arm and leg to match this movement. Each side counts as one repetition.

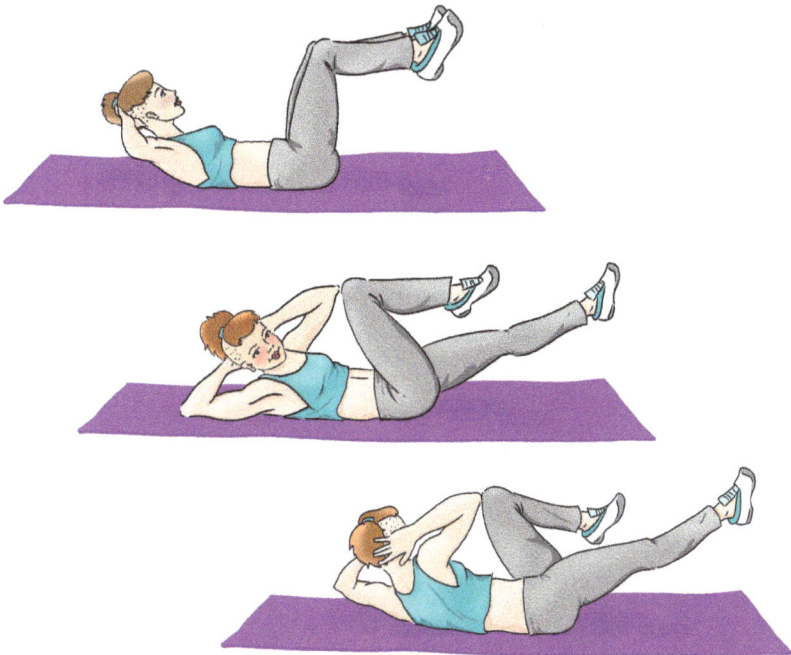

Seated knee tuck

Seated knee tucks focus on the lower abdominals.

Sit on your mat or towel with your legs bent and the soles of your feet flat on the ground. Place your palms down on either side of your hips, leaning back slightly until you can feel tension in your abdominal muscles (at approximately a 45-degree angle). Extend both your legs in front of you without touching your feet to the mat. Now bend both your legs back up towards your chest. This is one repetition completed. Maintain your balance by using your abdominals more so than leaning back on your hands. Keep your core engaged.

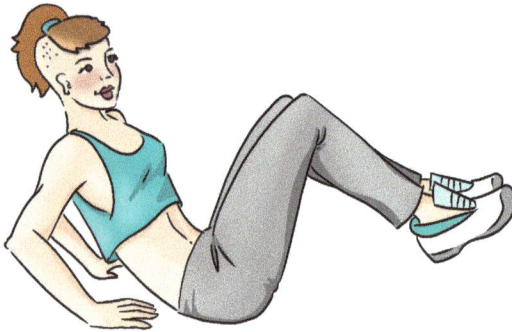

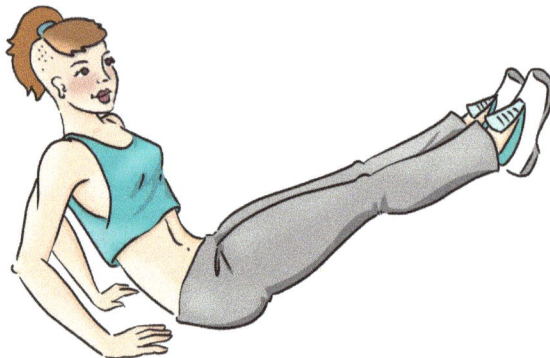

Scissor kick

This movement targets the lower abdominals, but it will also benefit your gluteal, quadriceps and adductor muscles, all of which build a strong core.

Lie supine on your mat or towel, with your legs extended. Place your hands along your sides – or, to provide extra support to your lower back, place them under your glutes – and focus on pressing your lower back into the ground. Maintaining contact between the ground and your lower back will engage your core. Lift both your legs, keeping your head in contact with the ground. Now lift one leg up while at the same time lowering the other one (at no time during the scissor kick should your legs or feet touch the ground). Alternate this up-and-down scissor action with your right and left leg. Each leg scissor movement is counted as one repetition completed.

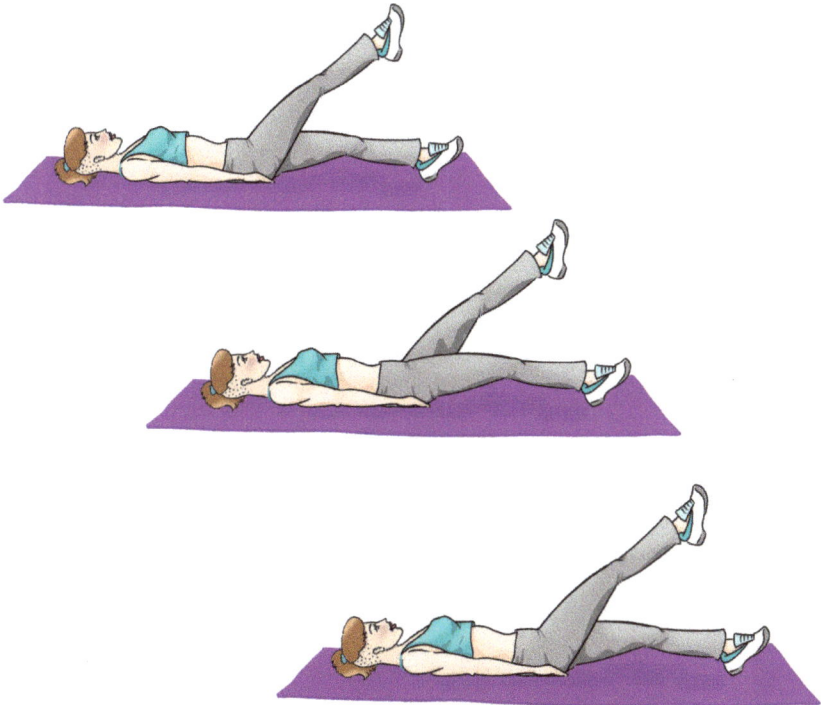

V-Up/Jack-knife sit-up

This is an advanced abdominal movement and it requires some practice, core strength, stability and balance.

Lie supine on your mat or towel, with your legs fully extended in front of you and your arms stretched out over your head. Simultaneously raise both your legs and torso off the ground towards each other, reaching your hands towards your toes at the top of the movement. Controlling the action, return to your starting position. This is one repetition completed.

During the movement, try to keep your legs as straight as possible, but if there is too much tension in your hamstrings (the back of your legs), you can bend your knees slightly.

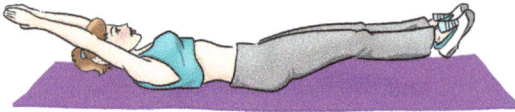

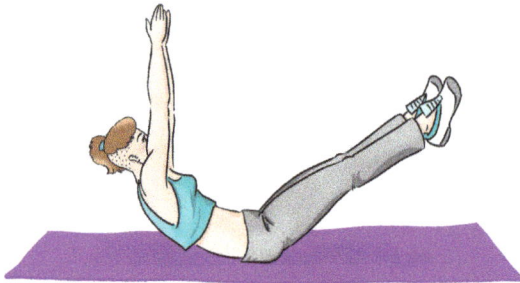

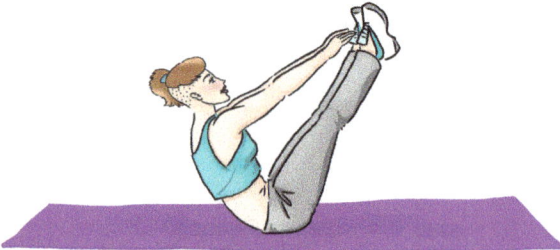

Single-leg V-up

This is a slightly easier version of the V-up.

Lie on your mat or towel, with your legs fully extended in front of you and your arms stretched out over your head. Now, simultaneously raise your right leg and torso and reach up towards your right foot. Controlling the movement, return to your starting position. Now repeat the action with your left leg. Each leg is counted as one repetition completed. Keep your legs as straight as possible.

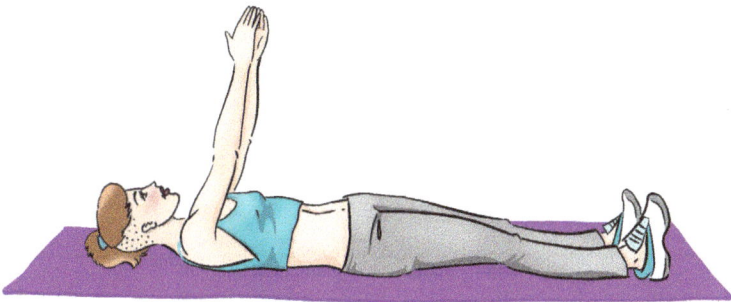

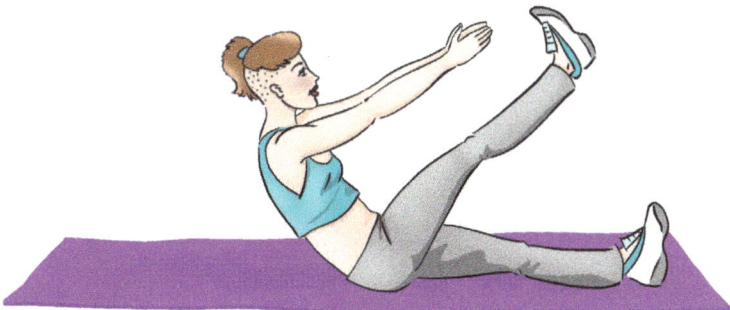

High plank

The plank is one of the best isometric strength exercises that you can do for your core. (Isometric strength – or static strength – exercises involve holding a position for a certain period of time rather than moving.) Depending on the plank you perform, you will also build strength in your shoulders, arms, glutes and legs.

Start by lying down as if you were about to do a push up. Place your palms on the floor next to your shoulders and flex your feet, with your toes and the balls of your feet pressed down on the floor. Take a deep breath and raise yourself into a push-up position. Holding the top of your push-up, your body should be in a straight line, from your heels to the top of your head. Draw your naval/belly button in towards your spine and squeeze your glutes/buttocks. Ensure your shoulders and shoulder blades are pulled down away from your neck and ears, lengthening through your spine. Look at the floor to keep your head and neck in a neutral position. Try not to hold your breath and instead breathe normally.

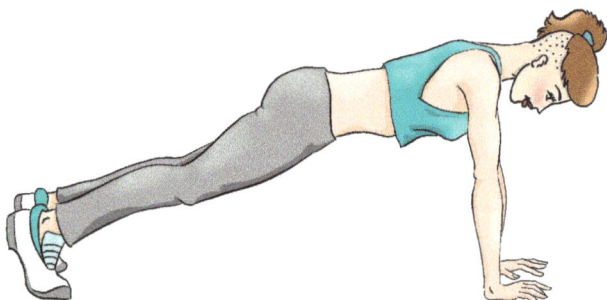

Plank on forearms/elbows

This is the most popular way to perform the plank position.

Rest your forearms on the ground, with your elbows aligned directly below your shoulders. If placing your palms on the floor feels uncomfortable, clasp your hands together. As with the high plank, as you raise yourself up, ensure your body is in a straight line and keep your core activated.

This form of the plank position can also be performed while resting on your knees (see second illustration). Again, just make sure your body is in a straight line and your core is activated.

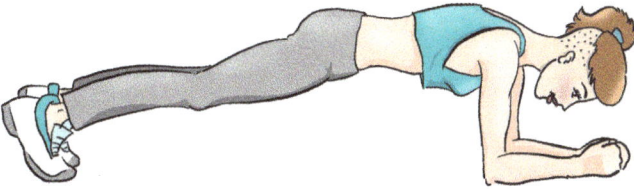

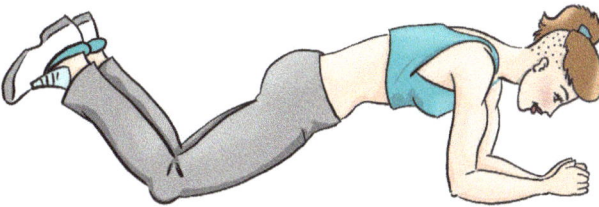

Plank shoulder tap

This variation of the plank position is a more challenging movement; its focus is on core stability rather than excessive movement.

Begin in the high plank position (the hands and feet position for the more advanced and the hands and knee position for beginners). Ensure your hands are directly under your shoulders, with your feet or knees slightly wider apart to provide a stable base. It is important to remain as stable as possible during this movement. To avoid unnecessary stress on your shoulders and lower back, brace your abs, squeeze your glutes and pull in your naval towards your spine. Maintain a straight line with your body and then lift one hand off the ground, moving it in a controlled manner to touch the opposite shoulder. Keep your hips square to the ground and avoid rotating your body as you lift your hand. Try to maintain a straight line and don't let your hips rise or fall. Alternate the movement between the left and right.

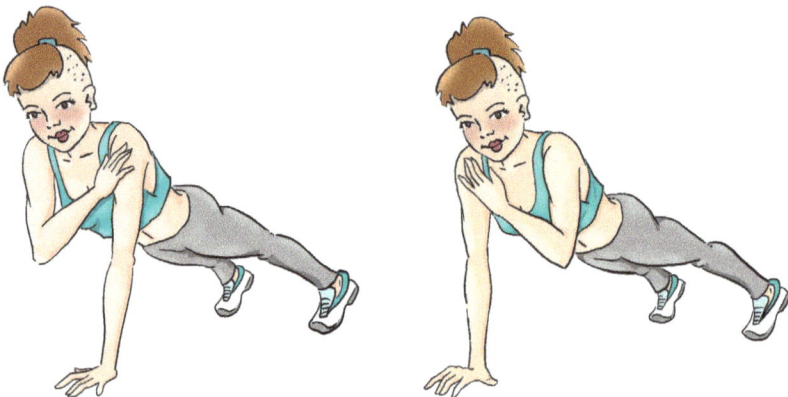

Plank toe tap

This movement will help tone and strengthen your shoulders, lower back and glutes.

Start in the basic plank position and alternate between moving each leg one to two feet to the side, tap the floor and then return to the start position. While doing this exercise, keep your glutes squeezed, your abdominals tight and your naval drawn inwards. Try not to let your hips rise or fall and keep the movement slow and controlled.

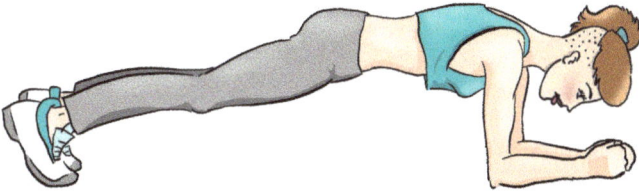

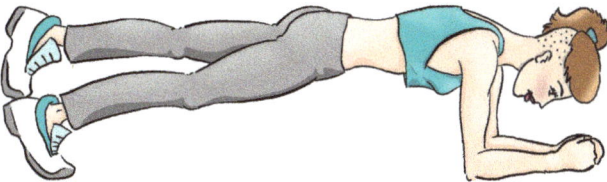

Plank walkout

This is great for core strength, and it will also challenge your shoulders, arms and chest.

Begin in a prone position on your mat or towel, resting on your forearms on the floor in line with your shoulders and feet. Now, push up, one arm at a time, into an elevated press-up/high plank position. Keep your body rigid during this transition. Ensure your movements are slow and controlled and do not drop or raise your hips when you begin to tire. Avoid the side-to-side 'wobble' of your body by keeping your core tight (squeeze your gluteal and abdominal muscles).

It is also easy to scale this movement by performing the plank walk on your knees. Pay attention to keeping your back straight, your core engaged and your movements controlled.

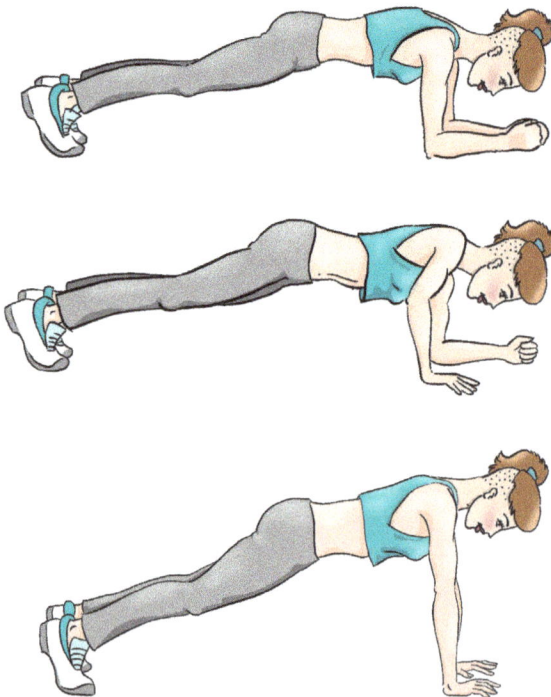

Side plank

This is great for strengthening the oblique abdominal muscles (sides of your abdomen). It will also build balance and coordination.

Start by lying on your right side, with your legs extended and stacked from your hips to your feet. The elbow of your right arm should be directly under your shoulder. Ensure that your head is in line with your spine, with your left arm along the left side of your body. Engage your abdominal muscles and raise your hips and knees from the ground, keeping your body in a straight line, from your shoulders to your feet. Focus hard on keeping your hips high off your mat and do not let them drop down. Start with a 20-30 second hold, alternate to the opposite side and repeat. Once you have practised this static hold a few times and gained confidence in maintaining the position, you can extend your top arm towards the ceiling, lengthening through your spine.

Scale the movement by bending the leg closest to your mat whilst still keeping your top leg straight and balancing on your elbow (see second illustration), the side of your knee and your lower leg. Once again, concentrate on raising your hips high off your mat, squeezing your glutes and keeping your abdominal muscles engaged. Start with holding this position for 20-30 seconds, alternate to the opposite side and repeat.

Please see images on the next page.

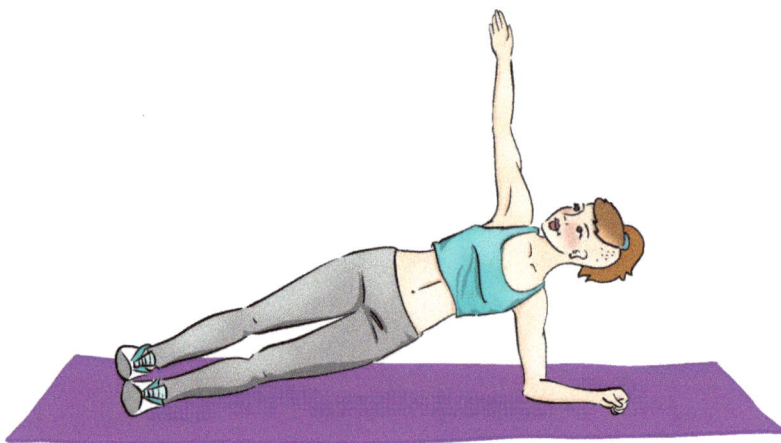

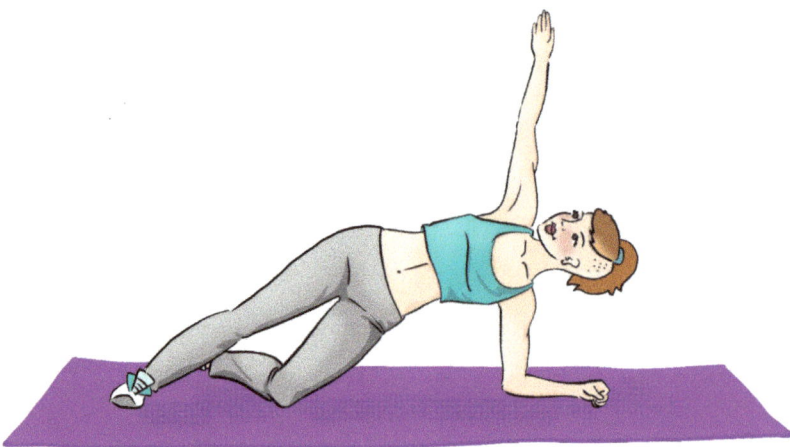

Russian twist

The Russian twist is another core strengthening exercise that targets your oblique abdominal muscles.

Sit on your mat or towel, with your knees bent and the soles of your feet flat on the ground. Lean back until your upper body is at approximately a 45-degree angle to the floor. In this position, your back should be straight (flat) and your abdominal muscles engaged (working). Interlace your fingers in front of your chest and, if possible, raise your feet off the mat, balancing on your glutes (advanced level). If this is too hard, keep your heels in contact with your mat and maintain a flat back and a 45-degree angle (beginner level). Now rotate your arms all the way over to one side of your body. Focus on rotating from your trunk/torso and not just turning your arms. Maintain your balance by engaging your core. Now rotate to the opposite side. This is one repetition completed.

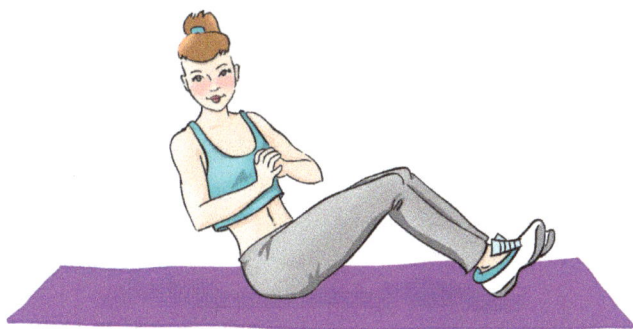

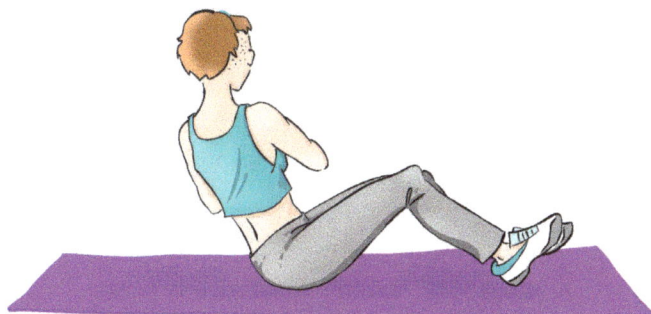

Russian twist continued

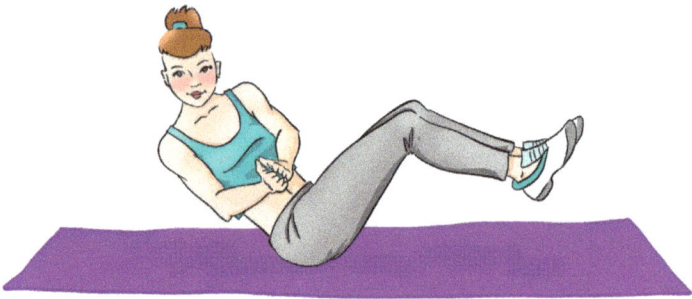

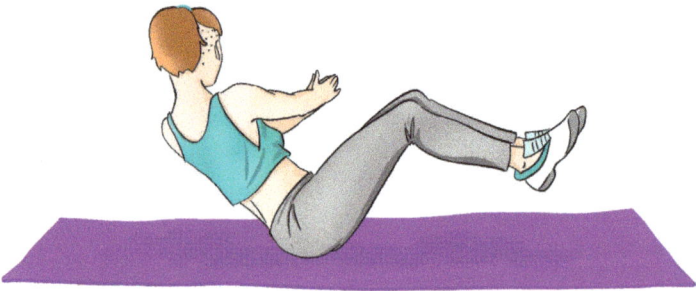

Superman/Arch hold

The superman, or arch hold, is an excellent strengthening exercise for the lower back.

Start the movement by lying prone (face down) on your mat, with your legs straight and your arms extended over your head or down towards your sides. Now raise your torso, arms and legs as high up from your mat as possible, squeezing your glutes, lower back and abdominals. Hold this position for 20-30 seconds and then lower yourself onto the mat. Repeat this action several times.

While doing this movement, ensure that you are looking down at your mat. This will prevent the hyperextension of your neck, thus avoiding a possible sore neck and trapezius (shoulders).

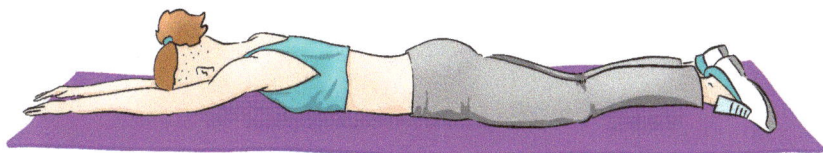

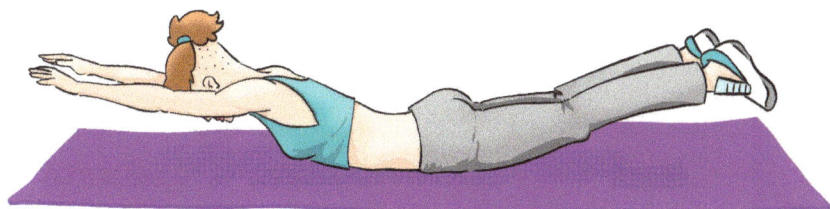

www.ingramcontent.com/pod-product-compliance
Lightning Source LLC
Chambersburg PA
CBHW041217030426

42336CB00023B/3377